Homoeopath
Exercise a

Emlyn Thomas
RSHom, DPhysEd

For my grandsons, Huw and Gareth Thomas

BEACONSFIELD PUBLISHERS LTD
Beaconsfield, Bucks, UK

First published 2000

Email: books@beaconsfield-publishers.co.uk
Website: www.beaconsfield-publishers.co.uk

British Library Cataloguing in Publication Data
  Thomas, Emlyn
  Homoeopathy for sports, exercise and dance. – (Beaconsfield
    homoeopathic library; no. 20)
  1. Sports injuries – Homoeopathic treatment
  I. Title
  617.1'027

  ISBN 0–906584–48–5

Phototypeset by Gem Graphics, Trenance, Cornwall
in 10 on 12pt Times.
Printed and bound in Great Britain by the Bath Press, Bath.

Acknowledgements

It would have been difficult to have completed a work of this nature without the help, interest and support of Veronica Fenn. I would like to acknowledge my indebtedness to her for being on hand to read and correct page after page of the manuscript, and indeed for making occasional kind remarks among the corrections.

I would also like to record my warm appreciation for the advice I have received from the following persons: Ilana Dannheisser, choreographer and homoeopath, Russell Davison, chartered physiotherapist specialising in sports medicine, Dr Fiona Dry, sports physician and homoeopath, and Dr Steven Kayne, community pharmacist involved in sports homoeopathy. Each of them made the time to comment in detail on a late draft of the manuscript, and I was very pleased to be able to take their thoughtful and constructive observations into account when preparing the final version for publication.

E.T.

Preface

This book is intended for all sports medicine practitioners, coaches, teachers, athletes (including games players and exercisers) and dancers who wish to use homoeopathic medicine. Many already do so, but in a limited way, relying on two or three well-tried remedies for specific acute conditions. It will also be of relevance for homoeopaths in their management of patients with sports, exercise and dance injuries. The material in this book will enable the user to expand his or her knowledge of this effective system of medicine, and to deliver a faster and more complete healing after injury.

Homoeopathy is simple until it becomes complicated, and I have done my best to keep it simple. It has been necessary to delve into the principles and background in order to help the reader understand homoeopathy in a way that is deeper than merely using a handbook to look up a condition and pick a remedy. This understanding will make the reader a more effective and confident prescriber.

The book is presented in two sections. The first explains homoeopathy and its development from a sports, exercise and dance point of view.

The second section looks at using homoeopathy to treat injury with regard to first contact, regional injuries and the common complaints that beset active people. With its descriptions of our remedies and a detailed index of conditions and remedies, this section can be regarded as a therapeutic handbook for choosing the best remedy. In conclusion, it examines ways in which performance may be improved.

Contents

Homoeopathy – A Basic Outline

Contents

Contents

Applying Homoeopathy

Contents

Contents

Contents

Contents

Contents

Contents

Contents

Advanced Uses of Homoeopathy

Contents

Introduction

When I worked on rehabilitating athletes, games players and other active people after injury, I often thought that there must be something more I could do to help them. Recovery often seemed frustratingly slow, muscle atrophy always seemed out of proportion to the injury, and my patients always needed much more motivating than expected – sports injuries patients were often difficult to deal with. We had to be careful not to upset them because they seemed 'touchy', fastidious, and very dissatisfied with their previous treatment. I did not recognise, in those days, how injury affects the whole person.

An injury of my own led me to discover homoeopathic medicine. I went to see my GP after a ligament injury and his receptionist suggested that homoeopathic Arnica and Ruta might help. I bought the remedies and took them. Immediately less depressed at the thought of being injured and inactive, I set about exercising, recovering and rehabilitating myself with enthusiasm. The injury cleared up wonderfully quickly and I was running and training again within days instead of weeks. I have no doubt that it was the homoeopathic medicine that stimulated my own speedy recovery, and I have blessed that anonymous receptionist ever since.

Homoeopathy treats the whole person. This book will explain how you, as a sports medicine professional, team manager, coach or dance director, athlete, dancer or individual performer in any physical activity, can use homoeopathy safely to heal your charges and yourself after injury.

The Injury Problem in Sport

Each year there are over nineteen million exercise-related injuries in the UK, more than half of them potentially serious. Of these, it is estimated that 1.4 million result in people having to take time off work, on average for six days. The estimated cost of lost work exceeds £400 million, and that of direct treatment for injuries £240 million.

1

It is not only the financial effects of injuries that are important. The injured athlete or dancer is one who no longer performs at his or her optimum level. And it is not only the professional athlete or dancer who is affected. The amateur who relies on exercise to keep fit, whether by a regular game of squash or football, jogging, aerobics or dance, suffers when denied this exercise through injury. His or her efficiency also suffers. Depression, dissatisfaction and lethargy set in, life is less rewarding and there is a loss of self-esteem. These may be associated with feelings of guilt at being less than efficient. The effects of injury on business, social and domestic life can be severe.

Dance Injuries and Treatment

If a dancer is injured there is no dance. Dance is a high-risk business, like all athletic endeavour, and the physical demands in both are much greater than ever before. When injuries happen, performances are spoiled, audiences disappointed and careers imperilled.

Fit to Dance, the report of the National Inquiry into Dancers' Health and Injury by Dr Peter Brinson and Fiona Dick, lists the following long-term aims:

1) To prevent or reduce dancers' injuries and illness.
2) To safeguard and prolong dancers' careers, by enhancing their physical and artistic wellbeing.
3) To benefit personal and dance company budgets through savings from improvements in dancers' health.

Many dancers and students have little money to pay for treatment, and this seems to be one of the main drawbacks to recovery. The temptation is to hope that an injury will heal on its own. The reality is that slow recovery and shortage of money lead to anxiety, stress and further damage to the dancer's health.

Fit to Dance also states that half of dancers in UK and two-thirds of dancers in Australia have chronic injuries, often sustained early in their careers, which affect their dancing

Dancers recognise – because of the unavoidable intellectual, emotional and mental element of their performance – that there is always a psychological effect of injury. This agrees with the homoeopathic point of view that injury always has a more general effect on the organism than the simply physical. A system of medicine that treats the whole person is especially appropriate for dance injuries. One that is also inexpensive and lends itself to self-prescribing also fulfils the needs of dancers and students. Homoeopathy is just that sort of system.

Homoeopathic Medicine

Little use has been made of homoeopathic medicines to speed recovery from sports injuries. This is because, apart from one or two remedies, little has been known about this powerful and inexpensive system of medicine among those who care for injury in the sports and dance professions.

A full range of remedies is available over the counter without prescription from many sources, mainly pharmacies and health food shops. There are safeguards regarding their use that the untrained user should be conscious of, and these are explained in the text. Within those guidelines the remedies are safe for anyone to use.

Basic Principles

The foundation of homoeopathic medicine rests on three basic principles. First, that injury – indeed any illness – is an alteration of the normal healthy state of the whole person. Second, that we can restore the person to their normal healthy state by giving them the smallest possible dose of a substance that would, in its substantial form, produce the same symptoms as the illness to be cured. Thirdly, that as homoeopathic remedies become more dilute, so they become more effective.

The Advance of Alternative Therapies

Unless they derive from research within a speciality, not infrequently funded by a pharmaceutical company, new concepts in medicine are not readily accepted. New dimensions were added to the world of orthopaedic and manipulative surgery by the use of, and competition from, osteopaths and chiropractors. Ideas from the field of lay practitioners are very much more difficult to accept, until popular demand overwhelms professional conservatism. Acupuncture and hypnotism are now breaking the barriers of professional orthodoxy.

Homoeopathy is close behind. There are now many doctors who use homoeopathic medicines to treat their patients. There are even more 'professional' (that is, non-medical but otherwise professionally qualified) homoeopaths practising their skills in response to public demand. Some GPs have discovered that homoeopathic medicine is so effective and economical for difficult and chronic cases that they employ professional homoeopaths in their practices.

Who Can Use This Book?

It is possible that you, the reader, will have already had some experience of using homoeopathy and some interest in alternative medicine. You may have used Arnica and Ruta to stimulate recovery from injury, and may have used First Aid books. These tend to over-simplify the system by suggesting that it is just a matter of looking up, for example, 'tendons', and finding Ruta. This will be successful for a small percentage of people, but will fail for many.

This book is more than a first aid manual. It offers a working background in the art of homoeopathic prescribing, and some insight into the way a trained homoeopath sets about choosing a remedy and managing treatment.

When a reader has become familiar with the contents of this book I would hope for the following outcomes:

- The sports medicine professional or trainer can use homoeopathy to deliver more effective recovery from injury and its consequences to patients or charges.
- A club manager, coach or dance director can help to maintain team, club or company performance by ensuring more effective recovery from injury.
- A sports performer, dancer, walker, fitness seeker, at whatever level, can use this book to help relieve the effects of injuries or overstrain, both for themselves and for colleagues.

Consult a Specialist

Although homoeopathy is effective for the treatment of sports injuries, it does not overcome the need for expert diagnosis and physical treatment of the patient. If you decide to use homoeopathic medicine to treat yourself, remember that you may be laying down problems for yourself in the future if you do not also consult your sports medicine practitioner for a proper evaluation of the problem. See Appendix I for details of where to find qualified homoeopathic advice.

How To Use This Book

Chapters 1 to 5 provide an introduction to the system of homoeopathic medicine, how the remedies are produced and tested, and guidance on managing the treatment. This is essential to the therapist who intends using homoeopathy seriously. There is much more to be studied and read than given here, and a reading list is suggested in Appendix III.

Chapter 6 offers suggestions on first contact treatment for injuries, and Chapter 7 gives some guidance for the treatment of overuse injuries. If this book does nothing other than convince you to use homoeopathic medicine for first aid after injury, it will have achieved a major objective.

In Chapter 8 I have tried to cover all the most common injuries, and suggest remedies appropriate to the common symptoms manifested in each type of injury. The reader may wish to look up the injury in this chapter, note the remedies suggested, and, if one of them obviously fits the symptoms, to use it. Failing that, for example, if more than one remedy seems suitable, check them all out in the Materia Medica in Chapter 10, and then select the nearest one to the patient's symptoms.

Chapter 9 suggests remedies for the common conditions that afflict sports men and women, exercise devotees, and dancers. There you will find colds, flu, tummy upsets and many more conditions, with suggested remedies. There are also suggestions for dealing with travel problems, heat, cold, altitude and many of the other conditions encountered by physically active people. Athletes and dancers tend to be more susceptible to these complaints than those with less active lifestyles.

Chapter 10 contains details of all the remedies listed in this book, together with some indication of their sources. Here we mainly consider the most appropriate uses of the remedies for sports, exercise and dance performers. There are many more aspects to all these remedies, and I suggest that the reader who wishes to pursue the subject further should obtain one of the complete materia medicas listed in Appendix III.

We explore new ground in Chapters 11 and 12. The former looks at the psychological effects of injury and remedies that may be effective in dealing with them, and the latter suggests homoeopathic means of improving performance. There is much more research to be done in this latter sphere, and I believe that it offers exciting possibilities.

Chapter 13 touches on other complementary therapies that may also be useful for treating sports and exercise injuries.

The book ends with three Appendixes plus a comprehensive general index covering all the conditions discussed in the book, together with a separate index of remedies.

HOMOEOPATHY – A BASIC OUTLINE
Chapter 1

Towards Speedy Recovery

'The unprejudiced observer, even the most sharp-witted one ... perceives nothing in each single of disease other than the alterations in the condition of the body and soul ... which are outwardly discernible through the senses. That is, the unprejudiced observer only perceives the deviations from the former healthy state of the now sick patient, which are:

1) felt by the patient himself,
2) perceived by those around him, and
3) observed by the physician.'*

Injury and the Whole Person

It is fundamental that when a physically active person becomes injured through trauma, overuse, or for any other reason, the normal healthy state of that individual becomes altered to a new, diseased state. This alteration of state is at once coincidental to the injury's onset, and unless we treat the person on all the levels affected by the injury, physical – mental, emotional and general – that altered state will continue to affect his or her wellbeing.

Homoeopathic medicine can be used effectively to heal the purely local effects of injury. It will reduce the swelling and bruising, relieve the pain and, together with the appropriate physical treatment, return a performer to full function sooner than without it. Because homoeopathy works on all levels of the person, in other words as a vitalistic medicine, it will also deal with the effect of the injury on the performer as a total organism, restoring the mental, emotional and general state of the individual to that of a fit and healthy individual. Recovery will be faster and more complete.

*Organon of the Medical Art, Hahnemann, trans. O'Reilly.

The Healer Within

When someone is ill or injured, his organism is 'detuned' like a piano or other finely-tuned instrument which has been damaged. The resulting dissonance makes it impossible to play melodies, or to harmonise with itself or other musical instruments. The 'sick' or 'diseased' instrument requires a tuner who will come along, repair any broken parts and retune it. The 'tuner' for a living organism is within that same organism.

Unlike a machine or instrument, the body repairs itself and performs its functions independently, carrying within it its own 'tuner'. Ancient medicine recognised the power of the body to control disease and called it, in Latin, 'vis medicatrix naturae' – the healing power of nature. This vital function is part of the life force itself, which Hahnemann (see Chapter 3) called the 'Vital Force'. Injury or disease disturbs this force. The correct homoeopathic remedy stimulates it and retunes the body to a recovered state.

As the following case illustrates, this retuning process promotes both recovery from the injury and a more positive mental attitude.

CASE 1

Eddy is a 23-year-old county standard rugby prop forward. He is a sheep farmer by profession, and his normal attitude to rugby, and life in general, is enthusiastic, energetic and dedicated. His game demands a high degree of upper body strength, and as a prop forward his back, neck and shoulders are subjected to immense forces.

He consulted me for severe pain radiating from his dorsal spine to his right shoulder. It had been niggling him for some weeks and physiotherapy was not improving it. The pain was worse when he rested after work or after a match. Normally easy-going, the injury had made him irritable and depressed because it was going on for so long.

As a sheep farmer, his work involves much lifting. His rugby position also involves much lifting when scrummaging. He felt his back was getting weak. The pain was worse at night in bed. He was restless and slept badly. He told me he dreamed of playing rugby. His back was stiff and sore when he first started moving but eased as he continued moving about. He told me that if he could keep moving the pain disappeared, and that a hot bath also eased it. He showed most of the signs of needing the homoeopathic remedy Rhus Toxicodendron.

A week after his first dose of Rhus Tox. and more physiotherapy he was much less restless, depressed and irritable, was showing signs of a good recovery, and three weeks later was able to play again without suffering the resultant pain and restlessness.

Comment

Rhus Tox. will often be recommended in this book because so many athletes or dancers present with this remedy's symptoms after injury.

Sports medicine professionals see cases similar to Eddy's every day. They are typical of many people's complaints at the subacute or chronic levels of post-traumatic injury, as well as during recovery. Many older athletes or dancers and performers will report them too.

The symptoms I used to choose this patient's remedy are not those which would normally be taken into account in a sports medicine diagnosis. They are, however, typical of those used for homoeopathic diagnosis and prescribing. You will recognise the symptoms described above as those which individuals tell you about, often in conversation during treatment or when they first contact you. They represent the altered state of the individual from normal.

It was Eddy's anxiety, irritability, restlessness, depression and worries about how his work and fitness were being affected, that led him to consult a homoeopath. These are the 'mental and emotional' symptoms which often lead to the correct homoeopathic remedy.

Feeling better after a hot bath, physical restlessness, better from continued movement and worse when lying down are 'general' symptoms that also lead to selecting the right remedy.

From a homoeopathic point of view, the important symptoms are not the aches and pains but the changes from the person's normal state of health. These changes are physical, mental and emotional, and in the general state of the patient.

The changes from normal in Eddy were:

1) He was anxious, irritable and depressed about his recovery from injury.
2) First movement was stiff and painful.
3) *Continued* movement and a hot bath relieved the pain.
4) Rest is painful; sleep restless and disturbed, dreams of exertion.
5) Injury from overlifting.
6) Weak paralysed feeling.

Regardless of the part, joint or limb affected, how it has been injured, and even how far in the past it was injured, Rhus Tox. will almost certainly help to control or eradicate the pain and speed recovery of patients whose mental, general and physical symptoms match those which this remedy is known to cure.

Recognising the Symptoms

An experienced sports medicine professional will recognise the above signs and symptoms as common among injured sports, exercise and dance performers, and they are the sort of symptoms that commonly emerge during a consultation without deep and direct questioning. They may not seem to be directly related to the pathology or tissue changes of the injury, and for that reason may not be considered in the diagnosis or preferred treatment. They do, however, reflect the changed state of the individual resulting from injury, and to ignore them is to leave the patient's condition partly unresolved.

Two or three simple questions are all it takes to find out more about a patient's general physical and mental state. Simply asking a patient whether he feels better once he has got moving, and whether the pain is worse when he rests, could be part of the normal consultation process.

Matching the Symptoms to the Remedy

In Chapter 3 I explain how a symptom picture of each homoeopathic remedy is developed, by 'proving' it from clinical experience and the accidental use of the crude substance. All the characteristic symptoms of every remedy are listed in comprehensive homoeopathic materia medicas. (See also Chapter 10 for a short materia medica of the remedies recommended in this book.)

If the symptoms presented by the patient match those of the remedy picture, then regardless of the pathology, location or date of the injury the remedy will be effective in treating that condition. The important symptoms should include the mental and general ones. Amongst the latter we include sleep, response to heat, cold, touch, fright and shock and other stimuli.

For example, an osteopath colleague referred the following case to me for chronic and persistent back pain.

CASE 2

Margaret, a dancer aged 26, had been referred to a specialist and had then received chiropractic manipulation, acupuncture, osteopathy and physiotherapy over a period of ten years. The pain had begun shortly after a dance session during which she twisted her back. Even after such a long time she recalls that she had been shocked by the pain, that she had been very sore and bruised and could not sleep for a few nights. Her bed had felt hard and lumpy and she could not get comfortable. She despaired of ever being free from pain but insisted, when friends asked about her back, that she was 'OK'. Her first words to me were, 'I may be wasting your time because I'm fine really'. In answer to one of my questions she agreed that she was very afraid of anyone even touching her back because it might hurt. She agreed she was reluctant to be touched at all, and that she avoided touching people.

Two years before this consultation she had been in a serious motor accident and had been unconscious as a consequence.

Comment

The symptoms that guided me to Margaret's first remedy were:

1) Injuries from falls, blows, shocks, jarring, head injuries.
2) Sore bruised pains.
3) Insisting she was well when she was not.
4) Fears touch.
5) Sleeps badly, bed feels hard and lumpy.

I gave her one Arnica tablet to take that night and one the following morning in the 30c potency. (See Chapter 3 for a discussion of homoeopathic potency.) The result was that she became free from pain a day after taking one dose of the remedy, and remained so for some six months. She then needed a different remedy because she developed new symptoms.

This case is an example of a homoeopathic remedy, prescribed according to the presenting symptoms, effectively treating a very old injury.

Margaret's state of health was altered by the original injury. It was further changed by the motor accident. None of the subsequent orthodox treatments could reverse the fundamental change to her total organism. Only a homoeopathic medicine could achieve this.

Although there are over two thousand homoeopathic remedies, there are a few remedies whose symptom pictures tend to recur frequently among injured sports, exercise and dance performers. I have already mentioned two of them, and other common remedies will emerge as we progress.

Once you are familiar with the symptomatology of these common remedies, you will find you are able to use them for yourself and your patients with success.

Homoeopathic Symptoms

It is important to recognise that homoeopathic medicine takes account of, and considers as 'symptoms' all the changes that the patient manifests, including mental and emotional symptoms. You will notice this from the cases quoted in this chapter and others. For example, the rugby player told me he was 'depressed, restless and irritable', and Margaret said that she felt 'fine' despite being in constant pain, and feared to be touched or struck. Symptoms like these are often used to differentiate between remedies, and the potential user should be aware of them.

Characteristics that a person will consider 'normal' are also symptoms to the homoeopath. For example, being sensitive to cold, or heat, or noise, not sleeping well, or very heavily, underconfidence (or over-confidence), indecision, sensitivity and many other characteristics can be taken as symptoms if they represent a change from the normal state. They may have been present for some years, but become exaggerated or develop after injury in a way that produces a negative influence on the athlete or dancer's performance.

Acute and Chronic Conditions

In sports and dance medicine terms an 'acute' injury is one of sudden onset, as in a traumatic event such as a sprained ankle or torn muscle. A 'chronic' condition is one of slow or insidious onset as in overuse injuries, or as in acute injuries that partly heal but settle into a lower-grade and much longer-term disturbance of the organism.

In homoeopathic terms an acute condition is self-limiting, is not deep-seated, and given time will eventually clear up or resolve itself. Chronic disease, on the other hand, is more deep-seated than acute, develops slowly and is accompanied by a general deterioration in the person's health. Chronic disease may manifest itself in different forms and organs and inevitably affects the person on all levels. Homoeopaths believe that the increase we now see in diseases such as cancer, arthritis, asthma and mental illness are evidence of the long-term stresses that the individual is faced with, including chemical pollution, anxiety and other forms of stress.

Traumatic Injury

In acute cases, homoeopathic medicines can be prescribed according to the pathology, and these prescriptions are often effective in relieving acute symptoms and promoting recovery from injury. Such specific prescribing is an important part of the homoeopath's skill and should not be ignored. Many cases of traumatic injury will require Arnica, and it could be a routine specific first remedy in those cases. The way that trauma responds to Arnica still surprises me.

Later in this book I list the remedies that have been found effective for specific acute pathological conditions. Your own experience will enable you to discover their value.

Homoeopathic Case-Taking

When a case is referred to a homoeopath he or she could spend up to one and a half hours taking the case history. The homoeopath's task is similar to that of a detective, but in this case one is looking for clues to the correct remedy picture displayed in the patient's present state, and how those differ from the normal state of health. The more pronounced the symptoms the better. Symptoms that are peculiar and characteristic to the patient are important, as are those that are strange and unusual. A burning pain relieved by heat is an example of a 'strange' symptom.

If a patient is unsure of his symptoms and needs much help to bring them out, they may not actually be of much use. Spontaneous symptoms are much more important. Even the fact that a patient cannot talk about himself may be relevant as a symptom.

As already discussed, the homoeopath will concentrate on mental, emotional and general symptoms more than physical conditions. It is an essential tenet of homoeopathic treatment that by prescribing a remedy which enables the central control of the organism to right itself, the acute symptoms will automatically and speedily be healed. Every injury, traumatic or otherwise, alters the central state of the individual, and that altered central state is demonstrated by changes in the individual's emotions, mental and general state.

Just as the purely physical effects of injury are worse in highly trained athletes because of the greater vascularity of their tissue, so the successful athlete or dancer suffers more serious mental, emotional and general effects from injury. These effects are not merely associated with the loss of function from injury, but can become much more deeply-seated. Anxiety from the loss of livelihood and ambition, depression and dissatisfaction are serious affects of injury. If these effects are ignored and left untreated, the long-term results may well be disastrous.

Common Symptoms

Certain symptoms are present in specific conditions. For example, if someone has sprained an ankle you would expect them to say that they had pain there, just as someone with arthritis or tendinitis will experience pain and stiffness. In homoeopathic terms these are *common* symptoms experienced by everyone with that condition. It is the difference between one person's pain and another's that the homoeopath is looking for. This is why we concentrate on sensations, location, concomitants and modalities, and search for the symptoms which are peculiar to that person.

The homoeopath will concentrate on the strongest and most important symptoms in the search for the matching remedies. He will divide the symptoms into mental, emotional, general and physical categories, and allocate importance to them as determined by the case-taking process.

Observation

Observations, first impressions and talking to others such as family members or the primary therapist, are important and I always pay much attention to them. I write everything down. Dress, posture, gestures, the way they speak and answer questions, colouring, and whether they are pale or ruddy are just a few of the details that appear in my case notes. These are comprehensive and as complete as possible, and are analysed by the homoeopath later, giving more importance to some symptoms according to how the patient reported them or how strongly they were experienced.

The Constitution

The concept of 'constitution' is a very old one, pre-dating homoeopathy. It is also a Victorian medical concept which has been carried forward into modern homoeopathy.

We regard the constitution as the physiological canvas on which the psychological activities of life are painted and enacted. It is the physical carrier of the life or 'vital' force, and the fundamental basis for expression of all the wishes and intentions of the individual. All the feelings of health, joy, harmony and love are expressed through the constitution, as are those of envy, jealousy, anger, anxiety and disease. The constitution carries the relics of past trauma, disease, grief and other influences, often going back for a generation and more.

The healthy individual's constitution is balanced and harmonised, and he or she tends to be at ease with the stresses of life and able to cope with modern living. There is a feeling of peace, health, relaxation and wellbeing. If the balance and harmony is missing, the individual lacks those qualities and may be at risk of not fulfilling his potential. There may even be a potentially dangerous situation, where serious illness or emotional excesses may result and interfere with the body's adequate or appropriate functioning.

Stress, anxiety, pollution, food, drugs, overexertion and lack of exercise are major factors which can stress the constitution. While we do not suggest that everybody is ill, we do believe that everyone has a level of susceptibility that makes it likely that they will develop certain symptoms or groups of symptoms when put under stress. These groups of symptoms may, in many cases, be recognised and diagnosed as diseases. They will almost always be recognisable as being similar to those associated with specific remedies. When there is such a recognisable similarity between someone's personality, mental, emotional and physical make-up, general attributes, likes and dislikes and other aspects of the whole person, and those of a homoeopathic remedy, that remedy is said to be his *constitutional* remedy.

If you find yourself faced with a sports injury or chronic condition which does not respond to your acute remedy, and you suspect it should be treated with a constitutional remedy, you should refer the patient to a registered homoeopath.

The Constitutional Remedy

The homoeopathic constitutional remedy aims to treat and resolve the imbalance and disharmony that undermine constitutional health. In theory there is no disease that cannot be treated with the correct constitutional remedy. Caution, however, is advisable. Treating serious, deep-seated pathology is not in the realm of this book, nor should it be attempted without the backing of a medical practitioner.

Just as everyone has a constitution, so the homoeopathic materia medica has a remedy that fits that constitution. There are about a hundred remedies whose pictures come up fairly regularly, and twenty that are prescribed frequently. Those twenty are what we call 'polychrests' – remedies whose pictures arise frequently and which have a very wide spectrum of action on all levels.

Although this book is mainly concerned with the prescription of specific and local remedies, the role of the constitutional remedy should not be ignored. Injury affects the constitution and its harmony. The specific, local remedy can restore the balance after injury, but more detailed evaluation by a homoeopathic specialist should always remain an option.

I recommend that you obtain a simple and clear materia medica and learn the pictures of some of the more common polychrests. A starting list should include; Argentum Nitricum, Aconite, Arsenicum Album, Aurum Metallicum, Bryonia, Calcarea Carbonica, Causticum, Graphites, Hypericum, Ignatia, Kali Carbonicum, Lycopodium, Mercurius Solubilis, Natrum Muriaticum, Nux Vomica, Phosphorus, Pulsatilla, Rhus Toxicodendron, Ruta Graveolens, Silica and Sulphur.

Safety

Homoeopathic remedies are safe for anyone to use and many thousands of people self-prescribe them. Most major high street pharmacies have introduced a comprehensive range of remedies in their shops. Apart from the chance that a very sensitive person may produce a short-lived reaction, homoeopathic remedies have no side effects or contraindications, and cannot be overdosed.

Repeatedly taking one remedy over a long period of time is not recommended. At first the remedy relieves the symptoms, but when the person persists in taking it over several months, say three times a day, the original symptoms and others can return with some ferocity and the condition may then become very difficult to resolve.

Another possible distressing result of taking a homoeopathic remedy may be a short-term aggravation of the symptoms. Anyone using homoeopathy should be aware of this.

Limitations and Risks of Homoeopathic Medicine

One risk of using homoeopathic medicine is that it can be used by a performer in an effort to keep going and thereby delay getting professional help. Every athlete, player, dancer, coach and manager should be aware of conditions which need expert medical attention and the dangers inherent in delaying diagnosis and treatment.

Homoeopathic medicines are not miraculous cure-alls. They cannot replace torn ligaments, repair a damaged meniscus, or regenerate new joints or tissue after many years of deterioration. For some conditions, including many sports injuries, homoeopathic medicine can only accompany other medical care. For example, homoeopathy can speed up the repair of a fracture as long as the bones have been set correctly. It cannot replace corrective surgery when its need has been diagnosed.

Homoeopathic remedies can be used in association with non-steroidal anti-inflammatory drugs (NSAIDs), but should be taken at least twenty minutes apart. (My experience is that it works more effectively this way.)

Sometimes it is difficult to find exactly the right remedy; homoeopathy may then be said to have failed, when it is really the prescriber's failure.

Homoeopathy, or indeed any other medication or treatment, is unlikely to work effectively if the maintaining cause of the condition is not removed. Some of my patients expect me to cure their hacking coughs (and their children's asthma) while continuing to smoke heavily. Athletes expect medicine to cure shin splints while they continue to run on hard surfaces.

Your First Steps to Homoeopathic Treatment

You or your colleagues probably already use Arnica cream or oil to reduce bruising. If so, you have already started prescribing homoeopathic treatment. If not, try it! You will be even more pleasantly surprised if you give patients Arnica orally following a trauma, or even a simple fall.

The next step is to obtain a supply of a few remedies in tablet form. Arnica, Ruta Graveolens, Bryonia and Rhus Toxicodendron are four excellent remedies to start with. If you cannot find these in a local pharmacy or health food shop, you could order them from one of the homoeopathic pharmacies listed in Appendix I.

Learn the basic symptoms for each remedy as you read this book. These are listed in the materia medica in Chapter 10.

When to Use Homoeopathy

The new prescriber of homoeopathic remedies will probably obtain the best results by prescribing for acute conditions immediately following injury or first referral. In these cases it will be found that, for traumatic injury, Arnica will be the most frequently prescribed remedy. Rhus Tox., Ruta and Bryonia may also be used frequently where painful symptoms and discomfort are still present in acute cases. You may increase your range of remedies as you gain experience, but I would advise the early prescriber to stay with just those four remedies.

Arnica is described in more detail in Chapter 6. It is the most effective 'first contact' remedy. Remember to use it. Everyone should have some Arnica tablets available in the home, car or office, and especially in the sports bag and medical first aid bag.

Later chapters in this book give details of conditions and circumstances where homoeopathy has been and can be used. In sports medicine, the professional could use homoeopathic medicine for every patient and every injury and condition, the exact remedy depending on the symptoms presented. It could help to make your other treatments more effective.

Not only injured athletes or dancers can benefit. Homoeopathic medicines can be used to treat all illnesses and common ailments successfully. Chapter 9 outlines some of the common conditions and the remedies that can help to deal with them.

Homoeopathy in Conjunction with Other Treatments

Homoeopathic medicines work excellently together with physiotherapy, osteopathy and chiropractic, and often enhance these treatments. During rehabilitation the correct homoeopathic remedy helps to stimulate the patient's positive approach to recovery. If there is a painful reaction to certain treatments or manipulation, a remedy will often provide relief.

Apart from acute and chronic clinical treatment of specific injuries there are other situations when homoeopathy will help your patients:

1) After manipulation or other treatment to nerve-rich parts which could provoke a painful reaction, especially of the cervical or other vertebrae, one Hypericum tablet in the 30c potency will help the patient avoid pain.

2) Before operations, give a daily dose of Arnica 30c for two or three days. This will help the patient overcome the shock and heal more quickly.

3) If a patient tends to suffer from the after-effects of a general anaesthetic, a dose of Phosphorus 30c taken soon after waking will help them recover.

Chapter 2

Homoeopathy in Practice

Homoeopathy for Injuries

Despite the potential seriousness and long-term effects of some sports injuries, there are few orthodox medicinal ways of helping the healing process. Apart from analgesics to control pain, and non-steroidal anti-inflammatory drugs to reduce inflammation, there are even fewer effective orthodox drugs available to promote healing. Prescribed and over-the-counter pain killers and NSAIDs may be effective, but their use is limited and there may be side effects. They may also include banned substances which could lead to an athlete's exclusion from a sport.

To neglect the treatment of the whole person – by concentrating exclusively on the physical healing of the pathology – will allow all the problems generated by injury to continue to plague the individual and affect his or her future performance. Such a regime will almost certainly ensure that the performer or athlete will suffer the long-term effects of the injury or injuries more severely in later life – injury predisposes to further injury

Orthodox Drugs

NSAIDs may counter inflammation and are available 'over the counter'. Their use for longer than about 72 hours may delay healing in a traumatic injury. An athlete or dancer should only use them with care, and should not do so to permit continued performance by simply masking pain and inflammation – take them with great care. The most common side effects are gastric bleeding and asthma, and they can also induce an asthma attack in sensitive individuals. They are contra-indicated for patients taking medication for heart disease, ulcers, hypertension and kidney problems. Little information is available about the long-term damage they may cause to the organism. No athlete or performer should take NSAIDs to mask pain in order to continue playing or performing, regardless of the importance of the occasion.

A performer may sometimes use corticosteroids to suppress pain and continue performing. Their effect is to suppress the acute inflammatory reaction and to reduce the phagocytic reaction of polymorphs and macrophages. The most serious effect of such treatment is to delay healing and decrease the bulk and strength of scar tissue. They are sometimes useful in treatment of chronic inflammatory conditions, such as recurring tennis elbow and other conditions where a palpable knot of scar tissue may be tender. Tenosynovitis, peritendinitis, bursitis and synovitis, as well as other inflammatory conditions causing pain and impaired function, may also respond well to injected corticosteroid. There is no published research showing the long-term effects of these drugs, and I suggest they should only be used with caution.

The level of pain can indicate the seriousness of an injury and the altered state of the individual. Never ignore it or play, run, work or dance through it.

Sports physicians are easily accessible and can provide a skilled diagnosis. Physiotherapy is the most effective treatment for injuries sustained by physical performers. From the immediate application of RICE (Rest, Ice, Compression and Elevation) to exercises promoting rehabilitation, and including all the thermal and electrical techniques, the physiotherapist or osteopath are almost the only resources for the injured athlete. Although the physical relief of pain, easing of stiffness, reduction of swelling and haematoma, and mobilisation by manipulation or other means, all go a long way towards speedy and effective healing, they often leave the deeper effects of the injury untreated. Rehabilitation plays an important part in recovery, but is often cut short or neglected because of the urge to return to activity. Because homoeopathic medicine treats the whole person it often ensures more complete and speedier healing, and thus a quicker return to activity.

The Patient, Not the Pathology

Look at the patient as a whole. Observe the way the person feels and responds to the injury, as well as to you. You will also need to ask a few questions, and use your powers of observation on the person and not just the injury.

Whenever I see a patient who has suffered an injury, the site of that injury may be secondary to its effects. Whether it is an injured ankle, broken leg, torn muscle or concussion, my first few questions usually decide the first remedy. If the injury was the result of trauma, whether due to a blow, twisting, stretching or friction, if there is haematoma, swelling and bleeding, and if the injury is very sore and painful, the person feels bruised all over and says he feels fine, I would prescribe Arnica immediately.

I am often asked to prescribe for people with an acute condition. Regardless of the location of the injury, my first few questions are about the pain, when it occurs and whether it is improved or exacerbated by continued movement. At the same time I observe how the patient seems as a person – posture, general demeanour, hot or cold, restless, fearful, nervous, afraid to be touched or treated, and as many of the obvious symptoms as possible.

The symptoms decide the remedy. The three people below received the same remedy despite having different injuries.

1) The badminton player in Case 11 (page 61) who had injured his lower back and complained that any movement was painful. He also said that it became worse if he continued to move, so that he had to keep very still.
2) A rock climber who fell and fractured the neck of his scapula could not get out of bed or wash, because even the smallest movement was painful.
3) A recreational runner was diagnosed as having plantar fasciitis. The pain under his foot made him reluctant to put it to the ground or move it in any way.

They all told me that it was not only moving the injured part that hurt, but also the fear of the pain that prevented them from moving. Any movement was painful – even moving the eyes or talking. In all three cases the patients were able to move again more comfortably within minutes of taking Bryonia.

A weightlifter with intense lumbosacral pain extending down his leg had to keep moving all night. He called me to ask for something to relieve the pain. I asked him if, when he got up and moved around, the pain became better or worse. He replied that to start moving was very painful and that resting was even worse. If he could keep moving it was OK. This case responded well to Rhus Tox. It would have responded equally well wherever the site of the injury, because the whole person becomes restless and uncomfortable when he needs Rhus Tox, first movement is painful but continued movement relieves the pain.

Prescribe for the patient, not the pathology.

Questions and Observations

For most other remedies you will need to ask some questions as follows, and write down the answers:

1) How was the injury caused?
2) How are you feeling?
3) Can you describe the pain?
4) Is there any swelling, heat or discoloration?
5) Does heat or cold help or aggravate?
6) Does rest or movement help or aggravate?
7) Do their hands or feet feel cold, or hot?
8) Are they thirsty or not?
9) Are they consulting their GP at present, taking any other medication or have other medical problems?

Use your own powers of observation to help you:

1) Do they look happy, or depressed?
2) What do they say about recovery? Positive? Negative?
3) Are they irritable, want to go home?
4) Are they sensitive to touch?
5) Do they keep well away as if you may hurt them even more?
6) Are they restless and cannot sit still in the waiting room?
7) Do they sit or lie absolutely still?
8) Are they dressed for winter even in summer, or the other way about?

Take Time to Choose the Remedy

For an acute condition you may feel the need to prescribe a remedy urgently. As I say throughout this book, in my experience the most effective immediate traumatic acute remedy is Arnica, and you can give it in every case of trauma. You do not have to choose the longer-term remedy immediately.

When dealing with the results of sports and performance injuries you will normally use a small range of remedies for the more common conditions. You will find that you learn to recognise the remedy pictures of those remedies and, as you are carrying out your physiotherapy, osteopathy or other treatments, your mind will be working on the probable homoeopathic remedy.

The Effects of Injury

The immediate effects of injury to tissue are well known. Whatever causes an injury, a blow, twisting, tearing, stretching or friction, the immediate effects will be the same. Structural damage to the tissue, muscle fibres, collagen, elastin, capillaries, arterioles and venules will be sustained. Cell death follows. Then the enzymes that begin the healing process are released. Local bleeding, or extravasation, can continue for some time. Although the healing process depends on this extravasation and the biochemical changes it generates in the injury site, the physiological reaction is usually much greater than the injury's healing needs. There is swelling, inflammation and bruising which immobilise the joint or area. For the purposes of speedy recovery it would be best if these disruptions could be kept to the minimum necessary, without the resultant pain and discomfort.

Research has shown that any foreign fluid entering a joint capsule produces atrophy in the surrounding muscles, and that more fluid produces more atrophy. It is therefore advantageous for recovery if the extravasation into the joint capsule can be kept to a minimum.

Remember also the emotional consequences when an athlete or dancer is injured. He or she immediately becomes 'different', is isolated from the team, group or other athletes, dancers and performers, and is treated differently from his or her comrades. Dancers – students especially – are often accused of 'wimpishness' by teachers and colleagues, and suffer the effects of rejection and isolation. They are often faced with the anxiety of reduced pay and actual poverty. These effects on mental and emotional levels cannot be ignored.

Age and Fitness

A fit person will have muscular tissue that is highly vascularised and will produce more bleeding when injured. During exercise the blood supply to the muscle tissue is greatly increased, and more extravasation will ensue.

Older persons suffer more from the effects of injury. Intramuscular bleeding and haematoma formation is increased after the age of about thirty, and in middle-aged athletes a small tear or insignificant blow can cause a large haemorrhage. Older athletes will often complain that they recover from injury or trauma more slowly.

As Arnica prevents the excessive extravasation associated with injury, you could prescribe it as the first remedy for every traumatic injury. For older performers, and especially those undertaking physically demanding events of an extended nature, prescribe Arnica to be taken before, during and after every event or training session. This will help them to overcome the effects of strenuous exercise more effectively.

CASE 3

I was 61, and despite being very fit, had been diagnosed as having extensive osteoarthritis. I accompanied my son, Steve, on a walk across the Simeion mountains of Ethiopia. We covered 300 kilometres, and climbed 6000 metres in twelve days. The first day's walk was 33 kilometres and 1000 metres of ascent. Towards the end of the day I took one Arnica 200c which relieved my tiredness and gave me a boost of energy. When we reached our camp site I was exhausted, stiff and very sore. I took another Arnica 200c, and slept well, The following day I was entirely free of stiffness or soreness. We walked 250 kilometres in the next eleven days. Naturally I was tired at the end of each day, but there was no more stiffness or pain, and no long-term effects from this strenuous and demanding exertion.

Inflammation

The next stage in the healing process is that of inflammation. This may last from a few minutes to several weeks, depending on the fitness and age of the individual, the amount of tissue damage that has occurred and the immediate treatment given. The human body's immune system cannot differentiate between infection and the results of trauma. The characteristics of inflammation are more appropriate to stopping bacterial spread, and exceed the response needed to cope with the results of trauma.

If we can keep the inflammation to the minimum necessary for healing, it is certain that healing will be swifter and more effective. Keeping the disturbance of function to the affected tissue to the minimum can only benefit the individual and promote his wellbeing. The amount of inflammation present after injury affects the amount of atrophy that occurs in surrounding muscles. This further delays an athlete or dancer's return to activity.

Arnica has the effect of stopping extravasation at an early stage, and will keep the haematoma and resultant inflammation and atrophy to a minimum.

Heat, Redness, Swelling and Pain

Natural sequels to injury and inflammation are heat, redness, swelling and pain. These demonstrate that the healing process has begun, and may, according to the seriousness of the injury, serve to immobilise the joint, muscle or limb.

From a homoeopathic point of view, these symptoms will all help you to decide on the remedy to prescribe, and pain is usually the most significant symptom.

Pain is the result of sensory and emotional experience. It serves to prevent further injury, and is a reminder of the need to keep the injured part immobile to assist recovery. As with the body's excessive inflammatory response to injury, so pain often continues long after it has ceased to be necessary for protection. Muscle spasm, atrophy, postural accommodation and psychological responses all serve to make chronic pain a pathological condition requiring separate consideration.

In homoeopathy pain is considered in much more detail than it is in orthodox medicine. We ask the patient to describe the pain in some detail. For example, a pain in the knee could be aching, boring, burning, cutting, dislocated, drawing, shooting or sore. The type of pain, together with other factors, will help to decide the remedy.

Let us look at soreness as an example of the different remedies we could use to relieve it.

1) A sore bruised pain following trauma will normally require Arnica as an immediate remedy.
2) Soreness following an accident when there has been great fright, or after surgery or manipulation, may require Aconite.
3) A sore pain when resting, or on first movement which is alleviated with continued movement, will respond to Rhus Tox.
4) A sore pain that seems located in tendons or ligaments, making the patient depressed about recovery, will probably respond to Ruta.
5) A sore pain generated by any movement will require Bryonia.

You will have noticed that the remedy is prescribed not only on the type of pain, but also for other symptoms such as trauma, fright, worse at rest, and during first movement but alleviated by continued movement. In simple acute cases we try to prescribe for two, three or more symptoms that coincide to form a remedy picture.

Mental and Emotional Symptoms

There are certain mental and emotional symptoms which most practitioners in the sports medicine field will recognise in patients during the first few minutes or days after injury. These are:

1) A fear of being touched or approached, in order to avoid further pain.
2) An insistence that they are well and do not need treatment.
3) A feeling of hopelessness or indifference.
4) Disturbed sleep because the bed feels hard and uncomfortable.

Some athletes will come to you because they are determined to get well and resume their sport. Yet somehow they despair of recovery, and they may be irritable, impatient and cannot wait for treatment, or may even decide to go home before you see them. They want to be left alone and quiet. If at the same time any movement is painful, a prescription of Bryonia will be indicated.

Others may be anxious and profoundly depressed, especially in the evening or at night. They will be restless and unable to sleep because they have to keep moving the injured part. This, of course, increases the anxiety and depression. They have to keep moving the part because it only hurts at rest, or during the first movement; continued movement relieves the pain. These cases need Rhus Tox.

The patient needing Ruta will also feel depressed, but this time it takes the form of dissatisfaction with himself. He will tell you that the injury was, 'My own stupid fault' and will describe it in detail. The injury is commonly associated with overexertion. The pain is in the tendons and ligaments and is worst when lying or sitting. Lying on the back in a warm room, and rubbing the part relieves the pain.

The Importance of Feelings

Some people will manifest feelings and mental attitudes when they are injured that may be unusual for them and seemingly out of character. Unless these changes are taken into account, recovery is unlikely to be complete even if the athlete or dancer seems physically healed. Every sports performer experiences feelings, and these are naturally increased as a result of injury. Their normal emotions change as the result of the altered state that injury inevitably produces. It is important to recognise and treat these changes to effect complete recovery.

A former captain of the Wales rugby team recovered incredibly quickly from a broken ankle and was able to represent his country only eight weeks after injury. Early in his first game he had had a clear run to the goal line and the ball was passed to him. Completely out of character, he dropped it! – he had been watching the approaching tackler. In later matches there seemed to be something lacking in his game. His tackles were less effective and he seemed to be less committed to physical contact. Rugby demands more physical contact than most games, and this player was renowned for his commitment. Despite his almost miraculous physical recovery something was missing.

By now you may recognise some of the mental symptoms of Arnica – a reluctance to be touched and fear of further injury. This determined player's too early return to top-class rugby could be interpreted as saying he was well before he had fully recovered.

By virtue of their profession, dancers need to be more emotionally involved in their performance than almost any sports person. Feelings and emotions are part of their work. While tantrums and antisocial behaviour are generally discouraged by the group force, it is generally accepted that dancers are 'artists' and therefore, by definition, emotional. One must be conscious of the dancer's normal state and note the changes that result from injury.

When combined with the physical symptoms of the condition the following mental and emotional symptoms will help you choose the remedy:

Anxiety
Depression
Anger
Guilt
Dissatisfaction
Sadness
Irritability
Denial of illness
Protection devices and posture
Aversion to treatment
A tendency to contradict.

Chapter 3

The Principles of Homoeopathic Treatment

The Vital Force

Homoeopathic philosophy states that there is a force in each individual organism that keeps it healthy, acting as a balancing mechanism for the physical, mental, emotional and spiritual existence of that individual. Homoeopaths believe this 'Vital Force' to be essential to life. When the it is absent, the organism is dead.

In its efforts to counteract disease and restore the organism to health, the vital force produces symptoms. These symptoms are not the disease – they are simply the body showing how it is coping with stress. In the case of sports injuries, the stress is that of the injury and its occurrence – the results include the pain, swelling, inflammation and loss of function. These occur because the body is coping with the effects of the injury.

Homoeopathic remedies work by helping the vital force in its attempt to restore balance. They act as catalysts. The energy of the remedy stimulates that of the vital force and assists it. Unlike orthodox medicines, homoeopathic remedies do not weaken the body's defence mechanism by suppressing it. Not only will the correct remedy alleviate the symptoms and allow the patient to feel that life is flowing harmoniously and normally, but it may also have the effect of making them feel even better than they did before the injury.

The Origins of Homoeopathy

Hippocrates (c. 470 to 400 BC), the 'Father of Medicine', suggested there were two systems of medicine: the 'contrary' and the 'similar'. Under the latter system he suggested that whatever a substance could produce as an illness it could also cure. Country people retained the knowledge of 'similar' remedies throughout the centuries, whereas medicine forgot them. The common names of plants give clues to their medicinal uses: eyebright (Euphrasia) is a bright flower that resembles a bright eye, with a reputation for curing tired and sore eyes; comfrey

27

(Symphytum) is also known as knitbone, because of its usefulness for healing broken bones. There are many other examples.

Samuel Hahnemann

Dr Samuel Hahnemann (1755-1844), the founder of homoeopathy, was practising medicine in Germany from 1775. Appalled by the suffering imposed on patients by his contemporaries, he began exploring the possibilities of infinitesimally small amounts of what he termed 'homoeopathic' drugs. These medicines would produce the same symptoms as the patient was suffering, and cure them.

His first experiment is reputed to have been with Peruvian bark, or quinine (Cinchona). He was translating Dr William Cullen's *A Treatise on Materia Medica*, which included a description of Cinchona and its ability to cure malaria. Cullen attributed its curative properties to its bitterness.

Hahnemann was sceptical of that explanation and decided to try the remedy on a healthy person as an experiment, choosing himself as the subject. He took the usual dose and found that he developed many of the symptoms of the disease, including some of the subsidiary symptoms which sometimes accompanied an attack. He later repeated the experiment with very small and dilute quantities, and again developed the symptoms. He had discovered that the drug commonly used to cure a disease produced symptoms in him similar to that of the disease. This was his discovery of the remedy now known as China.

The discovery was very significant for the development of homoeopathic medicine. By observing the symptoms produced by a substance in a healthy individual it became possible to suggest the healing properties of that substance.

He experimented with other contemporary drugs and common substances in order to elucidate whether a general rule could be developed. After six years of work with many drugs he established to his satisfaction a law of medicinal action which he expressed in Latin as *Similia similibus curentur* ('Let likes be cured by likes'). Many more years of experiment and treatment of willing patients allowed him to publish his great *Organon of Medicine* and *Materia Medica Pura*. He continued to practice homoeopathic medicine successfully until he died at the age of 89.

Hahnemann was a controversial figure in contemporary medicine, and his theories have continued to this day to arouse opposition and ridicule among orthodox practitioners. Despite this disbelief in the claims of homoeopathic medicine, ordinary people have turned to these methods in increasing numbers.

His astonishing results during epidemics earned him a reputation as an enlightened healer, and those results helped to verify his theory. His use of single remedies and extremely small doses dismayed the fore-runners of the modern pharmaceutical industry, and the apothecaries made his life in Germany so unbearable that in 1835 he moved to Paris, and practised there until his death in 1843.

Development of Medicines

When he diluted his remedies in a mixture of alcohol and water, Hahnemann discovered that the solution reached a level that no longer effected a cure. He subsequently discovered that if he shook the solution vigorously during the dilution process, it increased its potency and effectiveness. He used the leatherbound family bible, banging the bottle against it at each shake.

This vigorous shaking is known as 'succussion'. One explanation of the phenomenon is that shaking the diluted remedy releases its energy and imprints it on the liquid mixture. This method of preparing remedies by dilution and succussion is called 'potentisation'. Each repetition of this process produces a remedy at a new and higher potency.

There is still no accepted scientific explanation of the process of potentisation of a substance, nor of the method by which homoeopathic remedies work. Orthodox science cannot explain, and therefore cannot accept, how such dilute substances could have any effect.

Treatment with Similars

If healthy people come into contact with the poison ivy plant, from which the homoeopathic remedy Rhus Toxicodendron is made, redness and swelling of the affected part will develop with intolerable itching and burning. Great restlessness is worse at night, and when the person tries to rest. Pain, thirst and fever follow. Later on, rheumatic pains in the joints and soreness in the muscles develop. There will be painful stiffness in the lumbar region and the legs and arms become numb, with mental confusion, anxiety, restlessness and ill-humour. They will feel worse at rest, at night and if the weather is wet, and better if kept moving and after a hot bath.

Under the homoeopathic principle that like cures like, countless patients displaying some or all of these symptoms have been cured by

Rhus Toxicodendron, irrespective of the name of the disease or original injury which caused the condition.

Differentiating Between the Remedies

As individuals vary, their responses to stresses such as injuries are different for each individual, and so are their signs and symptoms. Treatment should also vary according to the individual and his or her symptoms.

Consider the problem of kneecap pain, a common complaint among joggers, tennis players, footballers, skiers and veteran marathon runners. Hill walkers of all ages may also experience this condition, which produces pain in the front of the knee. It commonly originates during exercise and gradually gets worse as the exercise progresses. Alternatively it may develop after the exercise has finished or in the following morning. Characteristically the pain gets worse after being kept in one position for too long, and there is a sharp pain when standing after sitting, kneeling or squatting. Walking downhill or even down stairs make the pain worse. There may be swelling around the kneecap, and there may be crepitation (a grinding sensation) under the kneecap.

We could describe these as the common symptoms of chondralgia patella, and there are many homoeopathic remedies which have all these symptoms. Because there are so many of them it would be difficult to prescribe a homoeopathic remedy successfully for just those symptoms. A successful homoeopathic prescription demands more information to differentiate between the possible remedies.

The two following cases may help to explain how homoeopathic prescribing works, and demonstrate how I arrived at the prescriptions in each of them:

CASE 4

Anne is a forty-year-old, fair-haired, blue-eyed and slightly overweight woman. She had recently returned to aerobics classes. One morning, after a class the evening before, she started to feel pain under her right kneecap. She described the pain as a rheumatic soreness which she first noticed when she was sitting having coffee. The pain was worse on rising from her seat. She tried squatting but that made it worse. She felt her knee was weak enough to make her fall over when she walked, and going upstairs was painful.

She felt cold, and her feet and legs were chilly. She thought that standing around after the class and getting cold might have brought on the pain. She mentioned that she wanted to attend aerobics because her friends had commented she was overweight, and she felt bad about it.

Comment
My prescription was for Calcarea Carbonica 30c, one tablet twice a day for three days, and I referred her back to her physiotherapist for treatment and exercise. The pain eased within a day. She started static quadriceps exercises to strengthen her muscles, and returned to her class two weeks later.

CASE 5
William is aged 40 and a keen mountaineer. He is a hard-working executive who lives a very full life – he works hard and plays hard. He began to suffer pain under his left kneecap when walking downhill. He woke very early the following morning, about 3 a.m., with the pain in his knee, and got up to find it was still very sore. It was worse when he rose from sitting. Standing was also painful. He described his knee as if creaking as he moved it, and his leg felt stiff.

Generally a warm person, he hated pain of any sort. It made him irritable. He became impatient with himself and others if he had anything wrong with him.

I asked him about his work and he told me that he was always busy, and that the worst thing at work was when people asked him questions.

Comment
William is a typical Nux Vomica type, and I prescribed this remedy in the 30c potency for 3 doses. I also referred him to an osteopath but he did not keep the appointment. He reported later that he had improved after two weeks rest.

A conventional diagnosis would have said both patients had the same complaint, and both would probably have received exactly the same treatment. Each received different remedies from a homoeopath, and both worked effectively.

Differential Analysis of Cases 4 and 5 (overleaf)

Differential Analysis of Cases 4 and 5

	Anne	*William*
Pain	Soreness. Rheumatic. Worse squatting and walking upstairs.	Soreness. Worse on waking in early morning. Worse after sitting. Worse standing.
Causation	Getting cold. After exercise.	Strenuous exercise in open air.
Sensations	Weakness.	Stiffness. Creaking.
Mental	Felt foolish when people talked about her.	Impatience. Irritability. Averse to questions. Enjoys working.
Temperature	Cold. Coldness of feet.	Warm.

Many of the symptoms described above are those of the whole person. For example – a sensation of weakness, impatience, feeling foolish, cold, warmth, worse after sitting. The approach in all such cases is to concentrate on the symptoms of the whole person, in other words, on their constitutional symptoms.

The remedy selected for each patient was the one that best suited their constitutional characteristics and not only their presenting acute problems. In other words, I treated the person, not just the pathology.

'Proving' the Remedies

If we are to discover which remedies are similar to a patient's symptoms, there has to be an experimental system for testing the remedies. Homoeopaths call this system 'proving'. Proving establishes the symptom picture of each remedy and allows it to be matched to that of the patient. Hahnemann conducted the first proving – of China, as already mentioned – in 1790. Since then homoeopaths have proved over two thousand remedies.

Hahnemann and his family and followers were so convinced of their theories that they were prepared to test their remedies on themselves.

They took small doses of poisonous or medicinal substances over long periods and noted all the symptoms they produced. Patients suffering from those symptoms were then treated with the potentised remedies made from these same substances, with very good results.

All the remedies used in homoeopathy have been tested on human volunteers, or 'provers', to elicit the symptoms they can produce.

The most common way of proving a remedy is to administer it to healthy volunteers using two groups under double-blind trial protocol. One group receives the remedy and the other receives a placebo. The remedy is administered in its potentised form, in various potencies. The volunteers record every detail of their physical, mental and emotional responses. Not all the provers manifest symptoms, but those who do have to be meticulous in the details they record. At the end of the trial the controller collates the records, and a remedy picture is built up in a form which has become common for all remedies.

The detailed remedy pictures are contained in the books of *materia medica*, and symptoms are indexed as 'rubrics' in reference books known as 'repertories'.

Clinical Experience

The symptom pictures of the standard remedies have been re-proved and substantiated many times. Clinical experience enables us to add new symptoms to these remedy pictures. We record symptoms cured by a remedy which may not have emerged in the original proving. Consistent cures expand the remedy picture by clinical experience. In this way, every homoeopath and user of homoeopathy can participate in developing the materia medica.

Accidental Provings

Accidental provings such as poisonings have become a valuable source of detail about some substances. Arsenic is one of the best known poisons and has been used for criminal purposes since the Middle Ages. Its symptoms are well recorded. In its potentised form Arsenicum Album is also one of the great homoeopathic remedies, with a very wide range of applications. I have used it often on expeditions to Asia when the sufferer has had discomfort in the stomach, vomiting, cramping pains and watery diarrhoea. These are also some of the symptoms of acute arsenic poisoning. The remedy picture of Arsenicum fills many pages of materia medica, and it is one of our most commonly used polychrests.

Another good example of an accidental proving is that of Gelsemium (Yellow Jasmine). Moonshiners used the plant to adulterate their whiskey, and some of the drinkers experienced symptoms of the central nervous system, including paralysis. They became heavy-eyed and shivery and their joints ached. They were confused and immobile, lying with closed eyes, but conscious. As a homoeopathic remedy Gelsemium cures symptoms of influenza when they include heavy eyes, shivering and aching joints and the person wants only to lie quietly, but not to sleep.

How Remedies are Made

Homoeopathic remedies come from mineral, plant and animal sources, some of them highly toxic. The first stage of making a remedy is to extract the mother tincture of the remedy from the original organism or source by maceration and steeping in alcohol.

Potencies are produced by diluting the mother tincture with a mixture of alcohol and water. There are two methods of dilution, producing two scales of potencies, decimal and centesimal, governed by the dilution ratios of 1:9 (denoted x) or 1:99 (denoted c). The number of such dilutions and successions determines the potency.

The mixture is succussed vigorously at every dilution. One drop is taken from the mixture at each stage and added to 9 or 99 drops of alcohol and water.

Although widely used in France and Germany and elsewhere in the world, the decimal scale is only used for a few potencies among English-speaking homoeopaths. Of these, only the 6x potency is commonly seen. This indicates that the substance is diluted to the level of $1/1,000,000$ or 10^{-6}.

The most commonly used centesimal potencies are the 6c, 12c and 30c. For these the dilution process has been repeated 6,12 and 30 times. The 'higher' potencies used are the 200c, 1,000c (or 1M), and 10,000c (or 10M). Some homoeopaths use potencies as high as the CM (equivalent to 100,000c). The point here is that the higher the potency the greater will be the dilution.

The following numerals in relation to the centesimal scale will be seen in the literature:

3c	which is a dilution of $1/1,000,000 = 10^{-6}$
6c	which is a dilution of $1/1,000,000,000,000 = 10^{-12}$
30c	which is a dilution of 10^{-60}
200c	which is a dilution of 10^{-400}
1,000c (1M)	which is a dilution of $10^{-2,000}$
10,000c (10M)	which is a dilution of $10^{-20,000}$

At 10^{-24} (12c) a level is reached beyond which there are theoretically no molecules of the starting material present in the potencies (the Avogadro limit).

Which Potencies to Use

Experienced homoeopaths take great care when prescribing the higher potencies. They are not generally suitable for home prescribing or for most acute physical conditions.

I tend to use the 30c potency for most acute, specific and local conditions. You should use the 6c or 30c potency for injuries, the 6c for first contact, and the 30c for later treatment. The higher potencies can have deep and long-lasting effects on the person's mental and emotional health, and may produce undesirable effects or reactions on those levels. There is also the possibility that repeated dosing with a remedy over a long period can exacerbate the very symptoms that it was intended to cure, and possibly also provoke other symptoms.

Use all remedies with care. As a general rule, limit each one to two or three doses and assess the changes after that. Stop as soon as an improvement begins to be evident. In the therapeutics section of this book you will find exceptions to this advice for specific conditions.

Whether to Treat the Specific Complaint or the Whole Person

As already stated, homoeopathy treats the whole person. It is essential to take into consideration all the person's symptoms. Yet we will recommend some remedies that you can prescribe and use routinely for certain specific acute conditions and injuries. These are tried and tested remedies that have always helped for acute conditions. Sprains to ligaments and tendons are known to respond well to Ruta, for example.

Is there not some conflict here? Remember that any specific condition affects not only the single injured part, but also the whole person. To treat any individual successfully one has to look beyond the 'presenting complaint', and beyond the acute injury to the 'totality of symptoms'. Some routinely given homoeopathic prescriptions for injuries are said to have 'failed' because they have not been prescribed according to the totality of symptoms.

How Can You Differentiate?

Here are some examples of remedies for trauma. You will see that they all have different symptom pictures. Each one fits a specific person as they react to the trauma. It could even be the same person on different occasions.

Aconite
1) After an injury or accident has a *very anxious* expression.
2) Will talk about the fright suffered.
3) Displays *intense fear and restlessness*.
4) *Anxious, excited, nervous and full of foreboding.*
5) *Intense* pain.
6) Arms and legs *powerless*.
7) *Chilled* before or during the accident.
8) Complains about the cold.

Arnica
1) Fears being touched, struck or approached.
2) Fears further injury.
3) Says he is well when he obviously is not.
4) *Very sore bruised.*
5) Symptoms of shock, dazed, coldness, fainting and/or confusion.
6) Better when lying down with his feet higher than his head.

Bellis Perennis
1) Deep trauma to soft tissue.
2) Cannot bear to be *touched* (much stronger than the Arnica person's reluctance to being touched).
3) Worse from a *cold bath or drink*.
4) Worse when *warm in bed*.
5) *Cold applications* ease the pain.
6) Following surgical operations to soft tissue.

Homoeopathic Help and Advice

Homoeopathy was recognised in the UK as an officially approved method of treatment when the National Health service was established in 1946. There are homoeopathic hospitals in Bristol, Glasgow, London and Tunbridge Wells, and an NHS Department of Homoeopathic Medicine in Liverpool. They all accept National Health patients, but are under some financial pressure because of the reforms to the NHS. Many GPs also practice homoeopathy under the NHS, although some are forced to confine their practices to relatively short interviews or to see homoeopathic patients privately. A list of homoeopathic doctors is maintained by the Faculty of Homoeopathy (see Appendix I). Professional (non-medical) homoeopaths are also employed in some GPs' clinics.

There are hundreds of professional homoeopaths practising in all parts of the UK and thousands under training at recognised colleges. A full list of registered homoeopaths (RSHom) is available from the Society of Homoeopaths, whose address is also in Appendix I. The Society represents the professional homoeopath in Britain, and works to maintain high standards in the practice of this increasingly popular type of medicine.

Chapter 4

Homoeopathic Symptomatology

Professional Assessment of Injuries

By now you will have some idea of what we mean by symptoms in homoeopathic terms, and you will realise that the term includes everything that you notice about your patient, together with what he or she tells you about their injury and themselves.

It is difficult to prescribe homoeopathic medicines successfully when a patient presents only one condition such as 'Tennis Elbow'. He may call it tendinitis, but for the purposes of homoeopathic prescribing such a diagnosis would be useless. By taking a few minutes to find out more about the condition, the patient and how he is affected by it, you will be closer to choosing a remedy.

Even if you have not made a diagnosis, as soon as your patient enters your clinic or reports an injury you will begin observing symptoms. He tells you what he thinks the problem is, you will have used your powers of observation and your experience to form an opinion of the condition. You will observe the patient's build, movements, posture, bearing and signs of pain such as facial expression or favouring a limb. The patient will also provide information about how the injury happened, or the action that caused it. He will tell you where it hurts and how it affects him.

You will then make a detailed examination of the injured part and inspect for swelling, redness, bruising and grazing. You will compare musculature, bony configuration and visible muscle spasm with the uninjured side if appropriate. Palpation will locate tenderness, its depth and precise position within the affected structure, and will elicit thickening, mass, scar tissue, induration, fluid, creaking or grating. You may be looking for crepitus. You will examine nearby joints, limb lengths and reflexes.

Common Symptoms

The above is the orthodox way to diagnose the effects of injury, and probably you use this method daily to choose the preferred treatment method. You will be looking for symptoms that make the condition similar to those you have treated in the past. Unfortunately, most of the symptoms elucidated in the orthodox way are, of necessity, common symptoms for common complaints and will be quite useless for homoeopathic diagnosis and prescription. As we have already discussed, the purpose of homoeopathic diagnosis is to differentiate between the totality of the patient's symptoms so as to enable us to choose the remedy most similar to that group of symptoms. We are looking for symptoms that make this person and his condition different.

To a homoeopath the name of a disease process and its classification are not as important as the collection of the patient's symptoms, because he treats the totality of those symptoms. An orthodox diagnosis of a condition and a sure knowledge of its implications, however, may facilitate the selection of the correct remedy, and is certainly not to be ignored or avoided.

Diagnosis

It is important that a patient should consult his or her regular sports medicine practitioner to receive a diagnosis of an injury or condition. At the same time, it is also possible to prescribe homoeopathically for a condition or injury using the homoeopathic symptoms presented by the individual, regardless of the conventional diagnosis or underlying pathology.

Observation begins in the waiting room, and develops as the patient enters the consulting room. An informed receptionist can play an important part in the homoeopathic diagnosis. Whether a patient is restless, whether he or she prefers to sit or to stand, whether they are irritable, impatient, anxious, very defensive against being touched, or they may seem depressed or very happy should all be noticed.

You will observe symptoms such as whether the patient looks pale, anxious or frightened, whether they prefer to be warm or cold will be evident from their dress. Perhaps they are hurried, nervous, or slow-moving and unconcerned, thirsty, need to urinate frequently, tense or relaxed, in obvious pain or stoic and unaffected. There are as many variations and combinations of symptoms as there are individuals. Fortunately there are only a few combinations of symptoms that seem to be common to many sports injuries, and arriving at an effective homoeopathic prescription for people with sports or activity induced conditions is usually quite simple and uncomplicated. Some of the common pointers to remedies are listed below.

If he or she is a long-term client you know well, you will already have a picture of them in your mind and will be able to recognise changes from the normal healthy state. These changes are the new 'diseased' condition generated by the injury.

Underlying Pathology

Occasionally pre-existing and underlying pathology may present as sports injuries, and the current injury serves to bring it out, in, for example, young persons with osteosarcoma whose condition presents as a fracture of the femur. Osteomyelitis, ankylosing spondylitis, Reiter's syndrome or septic arthritis may first become apparent through sports participation or injury. The correctly prescribed and administered homoeopathic remedy will often be effective in treating underlying pathology.

Rapid Traumatic Onset of Conditions

In most cases of sudden trauma you should expect to prescribe a dose, or course, of Arnica. Falls and collisions, however remote in time, will always respond to this remedy. Forcing, twisting, wrenching, strains and tears are most likely to respond to Arnica if it is prescribed within twenty-four hours of the trauma, but the effectiveness of the prescription will always depend on the symptoms, especially the mental and general symptoms manifested by the patient.

It is very safe to say that 98% of patients who have suffered traumatic injury, however caused, need a dose of Arnica to begin their recovery. It is also true that if they received a dose of Arnica immediately after the injury they would not suffer such long term ill effects of the trauma. Some patients may require Ruta, Bellis Perennis or Bryonia as a first remedy. (Refer to Chapter 10 for details.) Bryonia will often make painful movement easier and allow the person to begin active recovery.

Gradual Onset of Conditions

The onset of the condition may be gradual in dancers, runners, cyclists, walkers and other athletes, as well as in low-impact sports performers and exercisers. Allow the athlete or performer to describe the onset, when they first noticed the pain or swelling, whether it began with numbness or a particular incident of jarring, strain, or excessive exertion. Perhaps the person has recently increased the standard, amount or intensity of performance. Whether the symptoms appeared early or late in a run, for example, during rest or at night following exercise, and whether the symptoms are better or worse for rest are all important features to consider. There may have been earlier injuries to the same site. If so, you may wish to consider treating the relics of the earlier injury – it is important to consider earlier injuries to remote sites and their treatment. It is sometimes necessary to administer a remedy for earlier trauma before the indicated remedy will be effective, but I have found that the correct remedy will deal not only with the current injury but also with the remains of past injuries and even illnesses. The remedy that fits the whole person will also cure the whole person.

Recognising Homoeopathic Symptoms

It is helpful to divide homoeopathic symptoms into four classes.
- Location
- Sensation
- Concomitants (symptoms other than the presenting complaint)
- Modalities (how the patient is affected by outside influences, such as heat, cold, time of day, etc.)

You will find these classifications useful when you begin using homoeopathic remedies and are concentrating mainly on the physical and local symptoms.

Location

In most sports injuries the location of the injury will usually be very evident and obvious. Sometimes it is possible that the patient may feel pain in a location remote from the actual site of injury. For a homoeopathic prescription one takes the location of the pain as described by the patient, and notes it down as such.

It may surprise most people with an interest in sports medicine and injuries to find that, while the tissue involved, such as bone, ligament, muscle or tendon may be an important element in choosing the remedy, the actual location of the injury may be one of the least important considerations. In other disciplines the location is the first and most important indication, and certainly so for the injured performer. When choosing the homoeopathic remedy, however, the actual location of the pain itself, how the person feels and responds to his or her injury and environment, and the general condition of the athlete are often much more apposite.

Note whether the pain extends from one part to another, and use this

41

as a symptom. It is also important to note whether the pain seems to change its location, and what causes it to do so.

Sometimes you can find out about the size of the location, too. For example, the patient may indicate that the pain is the size of a finger tip, or perhaps smaller. The patient may indicate size with an outstretched hand, or grasp the part. Grasping the part may also suggest a sensation of tightness, constriction or grasping, which would be worth enquiring about. It can also suggest that grasping or pressure on the part relieves the pain.

Sensation

In the physical sense pain will be the most frequently reported sensation. This can present itself in many forms, and the actual sensation of pain felt by the person is important. Pain can be aching, boring, burning, cutting (or sharp), drawing, gnawing, pinching, pressing outwards or inwards, shooting, sore, sprained, stitching, tearing, or twinging. People are not generally able to describe pain, but sometimes use the above words to describe what they are feeling. In my experience, the most common descriptions of pain are aching, sore, gnawing, burning, and tearing.

Many people find it difficult to describe pain. Try it for yourself by asking your patients to describe the pain they feel after injury.

Numbness is a frequently reported sensation after injury. A patient may also report feelings of weakness, stiffness, heaviness, heat, cold, itching and tingling. Even if these are not in the injured limb, joint or part, note them and use them in determining the remedy.

A person may also describe a sensation of swelling. Even if there is no evidence to support the feeling, you can use it to choose the remedy.

Sensation is both what the patient reports and what you observe.

Your patients will describe other sensations: a feeling as if his arm were bandaged, or as if his legs were fragile. He may describe a cracking in a joint, crawling or formication in his skin, numbness, heaviness, of dragging in a limb, of weakness, of heat, cold and sensations of temperature, tension in a limb, or a combination of any of these or other sensations.

Interpretation

There has to be a certain amount of interpretation of the patient's description of sensations. For example, I have had a patient describe her head as feeling 'like a turnip', another described the pain in her leg as 'springing.' In both cases I had to investigate further by asking exactly what they meant. Many times, patients have denied having a pain, saying 'It's just an ache'.

Observation

You will observe some of the effects of sensations when you first meet your patient, in his posture, movement, whether he chooses to sit or stand in the waiting room, if he seems stiff on first rising from a seat, and in many other ways. You may observe that he is very protective of the injured part or totally avoids any possibility of being touched. You will probably do this naturally and automatically as part of your approach to your patient. Raise it more to a conscious level, and you will be embarking on a homoeopathic assessment.

You will notice heat or cold in a joint or limb, swelling, crepitus, etc., in your examination. Colour is also important. You should note these objective sensations in the case history, but they are less helpful in choosing a homoeopathic remedy than the subjective sensations reported by the patient.

Some Questions to Ask

1) Can you describe the pain and how it feels?
2) Are there any strange sensations in the joint or limb?
3) Can you describe how the limb feels?
4) Do you notice whether the injured part feels hot or cold?
5) What was the pain like when you were first injured?
6) How did you feel when you were first injured, and immediately afterwards?

Feelings are sensations on the mental level.

Concomitants to Injury

CASE 6

A colleague called me about the case of a footballer with pain under the instep, which my colleague suspected was a spring ligament strain. He had been treated with ice and ultrasound, and my colleague had given him Ruta. Response was slow, and we wondered whether the prescription was correct. I asked whether the patient was chilly, and the reply was that he was the opposite. He could not bear warm rooms, was worse on waking, and was much better when pressing cold things to his foot. Ruta patients are worse from cold.

On enquiring whether there were any other notable changes since the injury, I found that his abdomen felt very bloated and that he was passing a lot of wind, which was unusual.

I checked my repertory and found that there are three major remedies for 'Pain, sore, foot'. These are Lycopodium, Ruta and Silica. People needing Lycopodium often complain of feeling bloated and distended, and pass much wind. Lycopodium is the only remedy of the three that dislikes being in a warm room.

I suggested Lycopodium 30c, once a day for three days or until the pain was better. My colleague reported that the patient was free from pain the following day, and that subsequent recovery was swift.

Comment
In the above case, the first selected remedy seemed to be correct as a routine remedy for the location and sensation of the physical symptoms, but his 'concomitant' symptom of feeling bloated pointed to another remedy, which turned out to be the effective one.

During their provings homoeopathic remedies produced symptoms in different parts of the body and at different levels.

The concomitants are those symptoms, or changes from normal, occurring in other parts at the same time as the presenting complaint. It is rare for a person to experience a sports injury and feel sensations in only the injured part. The more serious the injury the more widespread will be the effects. The same is true of the long-term effects of injury; one never suffers the effects of arthritis only in the joint or joints. Sciatica often accompanies lower back pain. But what if the person also complains of cracking in his jaw when chewing? Or of feeling very sleepy after a meal? Perhaps you notice he is restless. There may be physical symptoms seemingly remote from the site of pain or injury. Appetite and thirst may be affected. They all form part of the homoeopathic picture of the whole person and are essential for successful treatment.

Always listen to what the person tells you about himself and how he had changed in response to the injury. Ask questions to find out about other changes since the injury. These concomitants to injury may be tiny clues, but are important.

Mental Concomitants

A patient mentions in passing that he has been sleeping badly since the injury. Ask why. Perhaps he has become impatient, or irritable, tells you he lost his temper. Note it and use it. Someone who insists that he is well when he obviously is not needs Arnica. Another who becomes very depressed and anxious when injured, and is kept awake by his injury, will need Rhus Tox. Someone who has become dissatisfied with himself and others, quarrelsome and prone to contradicting others when he has a tendon or ligament injury, will probably need Ruta.

Note whether a person is restless, fidgety, unable to sit, to stand, who moves from chair to chair and is so impatient that he cannot wait for the treatment to finish. Perhaps he is anxious about money, and how much your treatment costs. That too is a symptom you should note.

Note whether a person fears touch, or the treatment offered in case it may hurt him more. Note whether he is unusually cold, hot, sweating, red or pale-faced, looks frightened, tense and nervous, angry, guilty, absent-minded or forgetful. These qualities may emerge from clues in a person's conversation, and you can assume that they emerge because they are unusual or exaggerated as a result of the injury.

Physical Concomitants

Not only mental and emotional symptoms can be concomitants. Some injuries and conditions can depress appetite, others increase it. Some-times a patient may also complain of a headache. Extreme restlessness is a frequent concomitant of Rhus Tox. Shivering and backache are concomitants to the runny nose and sore throat of Gelsemium. To prescribe homoeopathic remedies successfully it is essential to know the complete remedy picture and to prescribe according to the totality of the symptoms. This is true even for treating acute trauma.

Modalities

These are the modifying factors associated with a remedy, like heat, cold, damp, dry, hot, time of day, movement, exercise, fresh air, etc. They may make the local condition, or the patient in general, feel better (amelioration) or worse (aggravation).

There are other important changes in the person that may point to a remedy. A person who needs Rhus Tox., for example, may complain that he feels much worse at night during wet weather. In Case 6 above the patient felt worse early in the morning. These are modalities. They represent changes in the person that seem to have little or nothing to do with the pathology of the injury or condition.

Closer questioning may have revealed that he felt bad-tempered on waking, when he first rose from bed, or after he had been up for a short time. All three are different modalities. Listen when someone mentions changes such as feeling better or worse at a time of day, before or after eating, in certain types of weather, in a warm or cold room, in bed, sitting, standing, walking. These can often point to the remedy.

There may be factors that alleviate, ameliorate or exacerbate the condition or symptoms. For example, locally applied heat may relieve a swollen, painful knee for one person while another cannot stand it, and cold may bring relief. Heat or cold in general (e.g. a cold room or a warm bed) may have similar effects, or may make a person feel better or worse in themselves. After a traumatic injury the patient may feel better when lying with his head lower than his feet. Body position can affect an injury. A person may feel worse or better when standing, sitting, lying or walking about.

The time of day can affect how a person feels. An injury may feel bad on waking, on rising, or at other times during the morning, afternoon or evening. It may be worse when lying in bed. The pain may wake the patient during the night. The exact time they are woken by pain is important.

Lying on an injured part may aggravate or relieve pain.

Recognising the Patterns

It is relatively easy to develop a technique of asking questions efficiently. After the first few prescriptions the patterns of most acute remedies become obvious, and choosing the correct remedy becomes easier. Occasionally you may find a set of symptoms puzzling, but a few minutes spent confirming the remedy in Chapters 10 and 11 will help you select the remedy that will best help. Fortunately, too, there is little danger in prescribing and administering one or two homoeopathic remedies in succession. They will either work or not, and there will be no risk of side effects or ill effects from prescribing the incorrect remedy.

Causation

Find out what caused the injury. If it was by a traumatic event such as a fall or collision, regardless of which parts of the body were hurt or damaged in the fall or collision, the fact of the trauma is important in choosing the first prescription. A fall resulting in haematoma, or abrasions, or stiffness, or even a fracture will probably respond very well to Arnica.

Arnica is the first remedy for an injury from forcing, twisting or wrenching, or if sudden force caused a strain or tear. You may then wish to consider other remedies that may be more specific to the circumstances. If the result was a strain to a tendon or ligament Ruta will almost certainly be required.

Even injuries that occurred in the distant past, sustained as a result of a blow, fall or collision will usually respond to Arnica as a first remedy, especially if bruising ensued. The patient will usually tell you about the causation because he or she has the event very firmly implanted in memory, and probably endures frequent 'action replays' in his mind.

'Never been well since' symptoms are very important as they point directly to the causation.

Maintaining Causes

Always be on the lookout for faulty technical equipment or training and practice conditions which may be contributing to the injury. These are as important for athletes as for dancers, and the informed practitioner will always be conscious of them when faced with overuse injuries.

Maintaining causes are circumstances that will continue to aggravate the condition as long as they are allowed to. For example, if shoes or boots are laced too tightly tenosynovitis of the dorsiflexor tendons can ensue. The condition will persist as long as the runner continues to tighten his laces too much.

Dancers are often faced with unsatisfactory rehearsal studios. Hard surfaces and unsprung floors lead to stress on backs, knees, ankles and feet. Dancers sweating heavily in badly heated and ventilated spaces can become susceptible to injury and infections. *Fit to Dance?* lists many potential causes and maintaining causes of injury to dancers, and recommends preventive measures for dancers and companies and schools (Brinson and Dick).

A Sample Case Studied in Detail

To give you an example of the differences between conventional and homoeopathic symptomatology it will be useful if we look at a case:

CASE 7

This young man was a 19-year-old athlete, a good squash and tennis player and a keen hiker. He first injured his knee at the age of ten when he fell and hit it against a rock. There followed some numbness in the knee for two days. The next occasion it troubled him was when it gave way three years later while playing squash. About eighteen months before consulting me he began to experience pain on movement and exercise, but continued to play squash at a high standard.

He had consulted his doctor, who had referred him to a physiotherapist for treatment. A partial tear to his left medial collateral ligament was diagnosed.

I observed that he walked with a limp in his left leg. Otherwise he was well built and moved competently. He said he had come to me because he was dissatisfied with the results of his treatment so far and depressed about his chances of recovery. His knee hurt when he was sitting down, and when lying in bed. Sometimes the pain stopped him sleeping, and he had to move his leg to find a comfortable position. I noticed he was restless, fidgeted and moved his leg often during the interview.

He described the pain as aching and stabbing, sometimes extending from his knee to his hip. Strenuous exercise made his knee hurt. Yet it was better when he moved it, when standing and when walking, except when he walked downhill after being in college all day. A hot bath relieved the pain. Cold wet weather made it worse.

He described himself as being 'fed up' with his knee and that made him very depressed. He could not concentrate at college, and disliked reading because he was dyslexic.

He liked sweets and sweet food, and added a lot of salt to his food. Tobacco smoke made him feel ill. He became irritable if anyone hassled him. His scalp itched enough to wake him at night occasionally. He sometimes had restless nights and dreamed of running or playing squash.

He also mentioned some abdominal trouble that recurred at intervals. He felt a sharp pain across his abdomen that made him bend over. This position relieved the pain. Watery diarrhoea followed, and was brought on by drinking milk or cola or missing his regular meal times.

Comment
We can use this case to see how a homoeopath approaches the assessment and treatment of a case, and arrives at a prescription.

After noting down the patient's symptoms the homoeopath usually turns to a repertory (as already mentioned, this is a reference book relating symptoms to remedies, under different headings known as 'rubrics').

In this case the pain was in his knee and extended up into his thigh. In my repertory of symptoms the only rubric that covered this symptom is 'Pain, knee, extending up the leg'. So I used it.

He described other symptoms besides those in his leg. He told me about his itching scalp, and abdominal pain followed by diarrhoea. He felt depressed and could not concentrate.

I noted down the locations of his symptoms as:

1) Left knee
2) Left leg (extension from knee)
3) Scalp
4) Mind
5) Abdomen

Sensations

He described the pain in his knee as 'aching and stabbing' sensations.

Aching pain in the knee was easy to find in my repertory, but 'stabbing' is not. I know from experience that it translates into either 'cutting' or 'stitching.' I asked him to describe it further, and he said that the pain was like something sharp like a needle going into his knee. 'Stitching' seemed the better rubric to use. Although there are 184 remedies listed for both those rubrics in my repertory, only 27 remedies have both 'aching' and 'stitching' pains in the knee.

He reported numbness in the knee following the original accident, and I used this as one symptom.

I observed that he was continually moving his leg as he sat talking to me, and noted it down as 'restless legs'. He also walked with a limp in his left leg.

Concomitant Symptoms

Although the presenting complaint was his knee, the other symptoms that arose during a thirty-minute consultation were important in helping to decide the required remedy. These were his itching scalp, abdominal problems and mental symptoms. Reading through the materia medica description of Rhus Tox. I discovered that the remedy also included an itching scalp, abdominal colic and watery diarrhoea among its symptomatology. It also has the mental symptoms of despondency, sadness and anxiety.

I included his mental and emotional and sleep symptoms as part of the case. Being depressed, dissatisfaction, despair of recovery, disturbed sleep and dreams of exertion are also very important symptoms of Rhus Tox.

Modalities

In this case the modalities were that the knee was worse when sitting and lying, and on first movement. Continued movement eased the pain. Strenuous exercise increased the pain. A hot bath helped to relieve it, but cold wet weather made it worse. It was worse at night, when lying in bed.

I could have found the symptoms in my repertory as follows:

Location/Sensation

Knee, pain, aching.

Knee, pain, stitching.

Extremities, leg, restless, night.

Concomitants

Abdomen, pain, cutting.

Rectum, diarrhoea.

Mind, despair of recovery.

Mind, sadness.

Sleep, restless.

Dreams, exertion.

Choosing the Remedy

Let us look at how I chose the remedy.

I took the following symptoms, when we find them listed in the repertory with the appropriate remedies they are called rubrics. By comparing the remedies listed under each rubric it becomes possible to eliminate many of them and to arrive at just one. This is how the rubrics looked in the repertory:

Location/Sensation

1) *Extremities, pain, aching, knee:*

Aesc, apoc, asc-t, bell, brom, bry, calc, calc-p, cann-i, carb-ac, chel, cic, clem, cob, com, cop, corn, dios, *Eug*, fago, fl-ac, gamb, glon, hell, *Hydr*, jatr-c, lach, led, lil-t, lob-s, lyc, lyss, mang-m, med, merc, mez, *Mur-ac*, nat-m, nux-v, *Ol-j*, op, osm, petr, phys, podo, ptel, puls-n, pyrus, **Rhus-t**, rhus-v, *Stram*, stront-c, syph, tab, upa, verat-v, xan, zinc.

Note that the remedies in each rubric are highlighted to indicate their effectiveness: bold type for the most strongly indicated remedy, followed by italic and lastly plain type for the less frequently needed remedies.

2) *Extremities, pain, stitching, knee:*
More than 100 remedies. Those appearing also under 'aching' include

 Apoc, asc-t, **Bell,** *Bry, Calc,* chel, clem, *Hell,* hydr, lach, *Led,* lyc, lyss, med, *Merc,* mez, mur-ac, Nat-m, nux-v, Petr, phys, podo, ptel, *Rhus-t,* stront-c, tab, zinc.

3) *Extremities, restlessness, night:*
Those included in the other two rubrics include:
Bell, Lyc, Rhus-t, Zinc.

Modalities

1) *Extremities, pain, knee, sitting, while:*
Agar, asaf, asc-t, aur-m-n, bell, calc, camph, carb-v, castor-eq, cist, coloc, crot-h, graph, indg, lach, led, mez, nat-s, phys, **Rhus-t.**

2) *Extremities, pain, knee, move, on beginning to:*
Led, Puls, Rhus-t, verat.

3) *Generalities, bathing, hot ameliorates:*
Anac, **Ars,** Hep, Rhus-t, Sil, Thuj.

It must now be evident that one remedy is outstanding, Rhus-t, and there are possibly two others worth considering.

The Prescription

Rhus Toxicodendron is worse from cold, rest, and beginning to move. The person needing this remedy is ameliorated by continued motion. He is described as suffering from despondency, and as being unable to remember the most recent events. You may know that the condition of dyslexia is sometimes said to be generated by a failure of short-term memory. Rhus Tox. also has symptoms of abdominal colic, making one bend double, and watery diarrhoea.

Even dreams of running and playing squash are listed among the symptoms of Rhus Tox. The materia medica describes the patient as having dreams of 'great exertion'.

He received two Rhus Tox. 200c, with instructions to allow one tablet to dissolve under his tongue before bed at night and on waking in the morning. I also recommended that he return to his physiotherapist for further treatment.

One month later he reported a great reduction in the pain and discomfort. Three months later he told me he was fit enough to enjoy his squash and college course. He occasionally experienced some pain after unusually strenuous exercise or a particularly hard match. His father told me his attitude towards college and his career had improved.

Let me stress that this patient only needed two doses of Rhus Tox. 200c to get better.

Mental and General Symptoms

So far we have concentrated on the selection of the remedy using main-ly physical symptoms. Even in the above case, what seemed at first sight to be a physical problem located in his knee had implications for the whole person. These had been ignored in his previous treatment, and his recovery was incomplete. So incomplete that this young man was on the point of giving up his sport and his chosen career.

The effect of the alteration to his central state of being was dramatic and critical.

What mental and general symptoms did the patient display which led to the selection of Rhus Tox. as a remedy?

The mental and emotional symptoms for Rhus Tox. include 'dis-couraged' and 'discontented', 'concentration difficult' and 'irritability'. It also has restlessness in bed, disturbed nights and dreams of exertion.

Dreams represent very strong mental symptoms, and I take special note of them.

I treat sleep symptoms as general symptoms unless the case is one of specific sleeplessness or waking. Disturbed sleep from the pain, and restlessness, are both covered by Rhus Tox. Relief from hot baths is another general symptom indicating Rhus Tox.

It is not only local pain in his knee or ankle, or anywhere else, that is felt when the Rhus Tox. patient begins to move. His first movements are all stiff and may be painful. More important, if he keeps moving he feels better generally, not just in the aching joint. Naturally that also feels better, but it is important to understand that the whole person dislikes the first movement, and is better from continued movement. You will see the Rhus Tox. patient in your waiting room sit for only a short time, if at all, get up and move around, and seem unwilling to keep still.

Given that same set of symptoms I would have prescribed Rhus Tox. for this young man whatever diagnosed condition he presented with, and it would have cured him.

Chapter 5

Managing Homoeopathic Treatment

When you have selected the correct remedy the next step is to give it to the patient. This may seem obvious, but there are ways of administering homoeopathic remedies that are peculiar to this system of medicine, and if you and your patient follow the system carefully the results will be more conclusive and effective.

Where to Buy Remedies

There are relatively few specialist homoeopathic pharmacies. I have listed a number of the major suppliers in Appendix I, and the various organisations also shown there will be able to provide the names of more local specialist outlets. Here you will find experienced pharmacists and staff who are themselves homoeopaths and who will be able to advise on prescribing and treatment.

You will also find homoeopathic remedies at most health food shops. The managers of these shops will often have a good basic knowledge of the most frequently used remedies and their pictures, and will be able to order higher potencies if you need them. It is also increasingly possible to find a good range of remedies at Boots and other large pharmacies, mostly in the 6c potency.

Taking the Remedy

Homoeopathic remedies are most commonly sold in containers of 125 or so tablets or pills. They are usually sold in the 6c or 30c potency. Higher potencies may be obtained from specialist homoeopathic pharmacies, or to order.

The patient should be instructed to take them as follows:

1) Take the remedy as indicated on the label by allowing one pill to dissolve under the tongue.
2) Take one pill morning and night/every two hours/as necessary/last thing at night.

53

3) Stop taking the remedy if you begin to feel better. Keep any remaining pills in case they are needed.
4) The mouth should be free from taste, so take the remedy twenty minutes after eating or drinking.
5) Put the pill directly into the mouth from the bottle lid and do not allow anyone else to handle them.
6) Store the remedies in a cool place away from strong smelling substances such as aromatherapy oils and perfumes.

I keep a stock of tiny envelopes for the purpose of giving patients a few tablets.

Rules for Prescribing

Some basic prescribing rules to follow are:

1) Give only one remedy at a time. In acute cases one should take one dose of the chosen remedy in the appropriate potency – that is, one tablet, pill or drop of liquid remedy.
2) If it begins to relieve the symptoms such as pain or discomfort immediately there is no need to repeat it unless the pain or discomfort return.
3) If the remedy has no effect after six doses, an alternative remedy should be chosen. The period of time over which you assess results will depend on you and the patient. It could be a few minutes, hours or days.
4) The pills or tablets should be allowed to dissolve under the tongue in a mouth that is free from taste; i.e. twenty minutes or so before or after eating, drinking, smoking or cleaning the teeth.
5) It is preferable if the tablets are not handled by anyone. Put one pill in the bottle lid, and then directly into the mouth. Or put it directly into the mouth from the packet.
6) Homoeopathic remedies must not be stored or kept near strong smelling substances such as perfumes, essential or aromatherapy oils or massage liniments.
7) Some patients can antidote remedies by drinking coffee, eating mints or even cleaning their teeth with mint toothpaste. I always recommend my patients to avoid coffee and mint for fourteen days when they begin homoeopathic treatment.

Frequency of Doses

Orthodox medicine has conditioned us to taking conventional drugs very frequently and for long periods. One dose of a correctly selected and administered homoeopathic remedy should be enough.

First aid and emergencies may require very frequent repetition of the remedy. I give one pill, dissolved under the tongue every few minutes until the patient begins to improve.

For acute, overuse injuries and other specific conditions give one tablet or pill, dissolved under the tongue, every twenty minutes for four to six doses.

The patient must stop taking the remedy as soon as they feel an improvement in their condition.

It may be that they simply forget to take the tablets as they get better. This is good sign of improvement and the effectiveness of the remedy. If no improvement is evident after four or six doses you should reconsider whether you selected the right remedy, and change it.

When Will the Remedy Work?

In acute, first contact cases expect the remedy to work immediately, or at least within a few minutes. I have known serious bleeding to stop in seconds after giving Arnica. As a rule, the longer the time that has elapsed between the trauma and the treatment the longer the remedy will take to work. The remedy should still work within fifteen minutes even a few days after the injury, as long as it was correctly chosen according to the symptoms.

In such cases, if the remedy has not worked after two or three doses it would be worth trying the next remedy listed in the appropriate chapter in this book.

For example, if Rhus Tox. fails to help the person who has sciatica down the back of a thigh, worse sitting and resting and especially in wet weather, it may be that a dose of Rhododendron will be better suited to his symptoms. This will be the case if the pain is rheumatic and tearing, and immediately better with movement and worse before a storm. You could stop the Rhus Tox. and start Rhododendron immediately.

CASE 8

A member of a group on a rafting trip down the Blue Nile in Ethiopia dropped a rock on his big toe. One guide had a homoeopathic first aid kit and gave him Arnica, but it did not seem to help much. The following morning the toe was swollen and very painful. The guide knew that

55

Hypericum was a remedy that helps injuries to nerve-rich parts, and gave him one dose. Relief of the pain was immediate, and the swelling reduced after two more doses of Hypericum.

Repeating the Remedy

If the patient suffers a return of the same acute symptoms he can decide for himself to repeat the remedy without fear of harm, as long as it is limited to five or six does. But see the case of the rugby player in Case 9 below, and always warn the person to stop the remedy as soon as an improvement in symptoms occurs.

Someone, for example, who suffers from a painful condition and has found a homoeopathic remedy to be effective may decide to continue taking it three times daily for some months, even though he no longer has the pain. This is part of the conventional culture and conditioning. Such long-term repetition could produce an accidental 'proving' of the remedy.

CASE 9

A 35-year-old rugby player had a long-term arthritic knee. After taking his case I prescribed Rhus Tox. and gave him one dose of the 30c potency. There was a decided improvement. Later he experienced a return of symptoms, bought some Rhus Tox. from the chemist and started taking two tablets three times a day as indicated on the container. He called me after a month complaining of a serious headache in his temples, so bad that he had to lie down, and his knee was bad again. I told him to stop taking the remedy and to drink a few cups of strong coffee to antidote the effects of the remedy. The headache was better a day later but his knee was still bad. I saw him again and prescribed another remedy.

Changing Symptoms

In some cases the person's symptoms may change rapidly. After a traumatic injury the athlete or dancer may at first feel shocked, bruised all over, and inclined to reject treatment. Arnica 30c, one dose every fifteen minutes, should be taken as a first contact remedy.

After an hour he may feel better, but even the smallest movement of the injured limb really hurts. He does not want to move, and cannot even be bothered to talk to anyone. Now he probably needs Bryonia 30c, and two or three doses will relieve the pain of moving. Later he may need yet another remedy as his symptoms change during recovery.

It may be necessary to change remedies two or three times in quick succession in urgent and acute cases as the symptoms change.

CASE 10

I was called away from my office to see a footballer who had twisted an ankle on our clinic steps. The person who called me reported that he had heard a 'sharp crack'. The patient was in serious pain, looked pale and shocked, and when I asked how he felt, said, 'Oh! I'm fine. Don't worry.' I gave him one Arnica 30c and referred him to the casualty department of our local hospital.

There was no fracture and a sprain was diagnosed. He was recommended RICE (Rest, Ice, Compression and Elevation) and was told he would have to rest for at least two weeks.

He had shooting pains up his leg that evening. Hypericum 30c helped those.

There must have been ligament damage, so the following day I gave him Ruta 30c to take once daily for three days. A few days later he said he had forgotten to take the Ruta after two doses, but was much better. In a week he was fully active again.

If the Remedy Does Not Work

Having chosen a remedy on the basis of the homoeopathic symptoms (rather than the conventional diagnosis), given it to the patient and sent him away full of hope that this new dimension to your treatment will be effective, you may find that he returns saying that it made no difference. For example the pain is the same, he is just as restless or uncomfortable and still feels despondent about recovery.

Something has gone wrong, and you may both conclude that it is homoeopathy that does not work.

It may not be homoeopathy that is ineffective but the prescriber or the patient. Perhaps the remedy was selected correctly but is working slowly and the results will emerge in a longer time scale than expected. Perhaps the remedy selected was not the most similar to the totality of the symptoms. Maybe there are underlying problems that require a different and more constitutional remedy. It is possible that your patient does not understand how to take the remedy, may be antidoting it or may not even have taken it at all. It may be that the bottle of pills, with the lid off, was left next to massage oils.

If a remedy does not seem to have worked you will not have done any harm or delayed the recovery. In that case there is no harm in changing the remedy and trying another. If a well indicated remedy appears to have no effect, do seek the advice of a qualified homoeopath.

What Can You Do?

1) Check that the remedy has been taken. That it was taken correctly. That the patient has followed your instructions. That he did not take it immediately after a cup of coffee. Try giving the patient one more dose of the same remedy and potency.
2) It may be the wrong remedy. Go through the symptoms again. Underline the ones that stand out clearly. Have you used those that are personal and individual to this patient? Check them in the repertory again, and read the detail of the remedies you short listed in the materia medica.
3) Have you missed something? If all your information still points to the same remedy you should assume that the remedy is simply working slower than expected, and give it a few more hours or days, depending on the urgency or severity of the condition.
4) You may need to change the remedy. If you then decide to change the remedy to one that is closer to the totality of the person's symptoms, you can go ahead and do so immediately with no ill effects.
5) There may be underlying pathology. If you suspect underlying problems you must refer the patient to his or her GP.

Storing Remedies

Store remedies in a cool place, away from direct sunlight and from strong-smelling substances such as the oils used in aromatherapy. When a stock of a remedy runs short it is possible to replenish it simply by adding unmedicated tablets to the few remaining in the stock jar and shaking them together. These will then become medicated by the original remedy.

APPLYING HOMOEOPATHY
Chapter 6

Traumatic Injury and First Aid

An injury due to a blow, or a series of blows, twisting or overstretch-ing, has the immediate effect of damaging the structural elements of the tissue. There may be damaged or torn muscle fibres, collagen, elastin and blood vessels. The amount of bleeding depends on the vascularity of the tissue affected. Muscle is more vascular than ligament or tendon and is more liable to bleed, especially during exercise when the blood flow is increased. After the mid-thirties intramuscular bleeding is much more profuse. In the middle-aged athlete and older dancer a relatively minor blow or small tear may cause haemorrhage. Older athletes therefore suffer longer recovery times after injury and unusually strenuous performance.

In joint injuries, although the synovium and capsule are not rich in blood supplies, significant bleeding into the joint may result from a rupture of a blood vessel within the capsule. As already mentioned, research has shown that this increases atrophy in the surrounding muscles. The more foreign fluid injected into the capsule, the greater will be the atrophy (Bentley).

Inflammation

Blood acts as an irritant and will increase the degree of inflammation. The greater the extent of the bleeding, the less efficient is the process of removing the cellular elements and fibrin of extravasated blood. Removal is essential before resolution and healing can occur. The more bleeding there is, the longer recovery will take. Conversely, if it was possible to limit the bleeding, earlier recovery could be effected.

It is important to minimise bleeding into tissues to reduce the degree of inflammation resulting from injury. An agent that reduces haemor-rhage would be an absolute boon in sports medicine.

There is one. It is Arnica Montana.

Controlling Bleeding and Inflammation: Arnica Montana

Arnica is mentioned very frequently in this book. It is the most important trauma remedy we have. I make no apologies for attempting to convince my readers to use it, because I believe it will speed the recovery of so many people. Keep it handy in every sports first aid kit, and also at home.

Regardless of the cause of the injury, Arnica will minimise bleeding after injury and its resultant swelling, inflammation and muscle atrophy. The effect of Arnica administered in frequent doses in the 6c potency as soon as possible after injury will be to reduce the effects of tissue damage. There will be less disruption of local blood vessels, and local bleeding will be restricted. Less cellular debris will accumulate at the injury site, and the visual effects of bruising will be reduced significantly. The healing process is made speedier and more efficient by taking Arnica orally. In the First World War all German soldiers carried Arnica and took it in the event of wounding or injury. There are so many examples of its use that Arnica can be recommended for first use in all cases of traumatic injury. The remedy prevents shock.

Arnica ointment will also reduce bruising, but do not apply it to an open wound.

Every sports team and sports facility first aid kit, every sports coach, trainer, physiotherapist, every aerobics teacher, and certainly every dance company, teacher and school should have Arnica available for use as immediate treatment after every injury, and use it. I believe this simple addition to first aid would be the most effective in expediting recovery of injured athletes and dancers.

Typical Signs

It would be useful to describe some of the typical symptoms of individuals who have suffered traumatic injury:

- When asked how they feel, they respond, 'I'm fine, OK, not too bad.' but do not want anyone to touch them, and withdraw from the possibility of further injury.
- They are reluctant to seek treatment, however badly they are injured. They feel very sore, bruised and aching. They may feel dazed, cold, confused and faint.
- They sit as if lost in thought, and want to keep warm.
- The muscles feel very sore, painful and bruised, not only where the injury is.

- They cannot sleep because the bed feels hard and uncomfortable.
- They want to be kept *warm*.

I could quote numerous examples of Arnica's effectiveness in stimulating speedy recovery from injury, but the following two cases may help to convince you.

CASE 11

A badminton player was running backwards for a high lob. He tripped and fell backwards, landing on his buttocks hard enough to send a shock up his spine and to feel momentarily concussed. The other players were very worried as he became 'grey-faced', and found walking difficult. I gave him Arnica 6c immediately, and advised him to repeat the dose every thirty minutes. He cycled home, a distance of about two miles. He described his reaction to the injury as 'very shocked at first, but the Arnica seemed to get me over that very quickly.'

He slept well. The following day, before getting out of bed, he took another Arnica. He telephoned me to say that he was afraid to get out of bed because even the slightest movement was painful. On rising extreme pain prevented bending and he could not put on his socks or bend to tie his shoe laces. This is a typical symptom for the homoeopathic remedy Bryonia, and I sent him a dose of it in the 200c potency. Movement became easier immediately, and he was able to dress and go to work. He experienced some uneasiness during the next few days but was able to play badminton and cycle regularly the following week. Despite my advice to refer to his GP for diagnosis, he felt his recovery demonstrated that his back injury could not have been 'very serious anyway'.

Comment

The Arnica kept extravasation, swelling and inflammation to the absolute minimum necessary for swift healing, as well as preventing the shock from a severe fall. It may also have reduced the effects of the concussion he suffered.

Stopping Bleeding

Arnica will stop bleeding from open wounds immediately if given orally as soon as possible. This is important in sports where a bleeding wound may prevent the athlete or dancer from continuing although the injury may not be serious. Epistaxis, or nosebleed, will usually respond positively to a dose of Arnica if it was caused by a blow. Another remedy may be recommended for epistaxis from other causes. (see page 193). If the condition continues the sufferer should seek medical advice.

CASE 12

A 23-year-old mountaineer suffered frequent nosebleeds, three or four times daily as a result of an old rugby injury. They became worse on arrival in India for an expedition, and during the approach to the mountain. He took one Arnica, and the nosebleeds stopped. There was no recurrence during the expedition, and no need to repeat the remedy.

Dissolved Arnica

On the rugby field I have used one tablet of Arnica 6c dissolved in a bottle of water, and have given a sip to any players who suffer an injury, especially one involving a blow to soft tissue. In many cases there has been minimal bruising and quick recovery. The efficacy of the remedy is not reduced by being dissolved, and it may even make the remedy more effective.

I strongly recommend routinely adding an Arnica 6c tablet to water bottles, especially for use in contact sports, or those where there may be some danger of injury from contact, such as rugby, soccer, basketball, hockey and boxing. Certainly dissolve one tablet in the water bottle offered to injured players. Using it this way may appeal to thrifty 'first contact' trainers, physiotherapists and coaches. One tablet can treat the whole team's injuries.

Preventing Fatigue

Arnica is an effective remedy against fatigue in strenuous sports or endurance events. It reduces the effects of injury and overuse. It generates renewed energy in tired runners, and taken before an event will help delay the effects of fatigue. The remedy has no side effects and its use cannot contravene any rules on the uses of drugs in sport. Refer to Chapter 12 for other remedies to prevent fatigue.

Older Players

Older athletes or dancers especially will find it useful to prevent the results of strenuous events being too painful or debilitating. Those returning to activity after a layoff will find it makes the process easier. Recovery is slower as one becomes older, and older athletes, dancers, performers or exercisers need more help towards recovery. See Case 3, page 23.

After Old Injuries

Arnica will work to help overcome the long term effects of trauma. The longer the time that has elapsed between the injury and the referral the higher should be the potency. For example, from one month to a year after injury I would give a dose of Arnica 200c, if the injury was between one and two years before, Arnica 1M may be effective, and I have prescribed Arnica 10M for an athlete who had damaged his cruciate ligaments five years previously. However, these higher potencies should only be prescribed under qualified homoeopathic supervision.

Other First Aid Remedies

Use Bellis Perennis if the person has suffered a deep injury and bruising with intense deep pain to soft tissue such as a blow to the abdomen or breasts. She will feel much worse if she becomes cold, and the pain may be so intense that it 'drives her to distraction'. In such cases Bellis Perennis may be more effective than Arnica. It is best to keep it as a reserve to give if the Arnica does not seem to work after one to four hours. Give it in the 6c potency at first, and repeat every twenty minutes.

Rescue Remedy (a Bach Flower Remedy) is an excellent first contact remedy for bruising and trauma if Arnica or Bellis are not available. A few drops of this remedy under the tongue prevents shock, and works in a similar way to the homoeopathic remedies.

Nerve-Rich Injuries

For injuries to nerve-rich parts of the body (see Case 8, page 55), such as crushed fingers and toes, Hypericum will be most effective. The pains are shooting, intolerable and excruciating. There will be some shock and any movement will be painful.

Hypericum is especially effective for relieving the pain of blows to the spine and particularly for falls on the coccyx.

Osteopaths, chiropractors, sports masseurs and anyone who manipulates the spine as treatment should know that Hypericum is excellent when patients react painfully to manipulation.

Head Injuries and Concussion

There are two main remedies that are both recommended for use after head injuries. Their use does not absolve you from referring the patient for medical assessment and treatment, but they may be used to speed recovery. They are Arnica Montana and Natrum Sulphuricum.

Arnica

Arnica prescribed in the 200c potency can help recovery and could prevent complications after serious head injury. All violent contact sports, especially boxing, rugby and association football involve the risk of serious head injury. After a head injury the blood from any intracranial haemorrhage collects and usually forms a subdural haematoma, or clot. Otherwise it may form an intracerebral haematoma if it gathers in the actual brain tissue. Arnica can work to prevent bleeding from damaged blood vessels sustained in the trauma, and could reduce the possibility of oedema.

Simply wetting the patient's lips with a solution of Arnica 200c could save his life, and will help him towards a speedy recovery by reducing the bleeding resulting from the injury.

Even if you do not have Arnica 200c available, use Arnica in any potency immediately following any head injury.

Arnica 200c should be available, dissolved in water, at every boxing, rugby or football match.

Natrum Sulphuricum

This person has a sick, crushing headache that is worse for noise. He suffers from vertigo, may vomit, and is irritable. This remedy tends to be more useful for the long-term effects of a head injury. See also Chapter 9.

Treating an Unconscious Player

Although you may be conditioned to avoid giving any oral medication to an unconscious player after a head injury, if there is a delay in getting medical help, an Arnica tablet dissolved in water can be administered simply by wetting the player's lips, and it will help. I have known homoeopathic remedies work when used to bathe an unconscious patient's wrists.

Give Arnica immediately on recovering consciousness, and routinely for anyone suffering from a head injury or concussion.

The special symptoms for Arnica after a head injury are;

- He says he is 'OK. Fine. No problems', and will not want any fuss, or to see a doctor.
- He may have trouble walking because of dizziness, may not even be able to sit erect, and is dizzy when he closes his eyes.
- His eyes may be bloodshot and his face ruddy.
- He will not want to be touched. He may show fear of being touched, and shies away from contact with people.

Resuscitation

Every coach, trainer, physiotherapist, manager, athlete or dancer and participant in any physical activity should know how to treat an unconscious person, especially one who is not breathing. The main purpose is to restore or sustain life until hospital treatment is available.

The British Red Cross and St John Ambulance training schemes are excellent, and every one involved in offering first contact treatment to injured athletes or dancers should seek their advice and training.

Homoeopathic Remedies

If unconsciousness is due to an accident, fall or head injury wet the lips with Arnica in solution.

If the patient is clammy and cold, almost lifeless, pulse imperceptible, not breathing, or the breathing is very rapid, shallow and cold, Carbo Veg. 6c may be used in solution to wet the lips or bathe the wrists.

If the unconsciousness is caused by haemorrhage, China 6c may both stop the haemorrhage and restore the patient to consciousness. Wet the lips with China 6c in solution.

Skin Wounds

Abrasions, gravel burns and similar wounds that do not completely penetrate the skin are common among athletes and dancers who train on hard or synthetic surfaces and matting. Foreign material must be removed to prevent infection. Wash the area with Calendula lotion, allow it to dry, and then apply Calendula cream. This homoeopathic cream will promote healing, alleviate the pain of the abrasion, and prevent infection.

Open wounds, such as lacerations or puncture wounds, are more serious. Arnica 6c, taken orally, will help to stop the bleeding. Do not, however, use Arnica topically as a cream or lotion on an open wound. Apply pressure to the wound and keep the part elevated. Refer the athlete or dancer for medical treatment if stitches are thought necessary.

Puncture wounds will respond to one Ledum 6c given orally.

Muscle Tears

Muscle strains or tears of whatever grade, as described by Fowler (1984) and Keene (1990), will produce bleeding into the muscle. The purpose of first contact treatment is to confine the bleeding and to limit the inflammation and swelling. The person should take one Arnica 6c immediately after injury and repeat the dose every hour for two days, or until the bleeding and shock reduce and he or she begins to feel better.

Follow the Arnica with Calendula 6c, three times daily for one week to promote healing, and apply Calendula cream or lotion twice a day.

Tendons and Ligaments

Strains and sprains to tendons and ligaments will respond well to Arnica as a first remedy. Follow the Arnica with a dose of Ruta to promote healing, alleviate the pain, and make the sufferer less restless.

Fractures

Arnica 6c should be given as soon as the injury takes place, or very shortly afterwards. It will prevent shock, stop bleeding, reduce bruising and swelling and promote wellbeing in the patient.

Spinal Injury

Any suspected spinal injury must be treated with utmost care and should be referred to a doctor as soon as possible. Everyone must be aware of the rules for moving people with possible spinal injuries.

Treat traumatic injury to the spine immediately with one Arnica tablet, or a sip of water in which Arnica has been dissolved. This rule applies to wherever the injury is located. It could prevent shock and reduce the long-term effects of the injury.

Refer to Chapter 8 for more remedies for spinal injuries.

Chapter 7

Overuse Injuries and Conditions

From 'Fit to Dance'
A senior artist with a ballet company had severe shin splints during his first two years of vocational training, probably due to being a late developer and growing very quickly during this period. While dancing in the corps he was identified as promising and pushed very hard. One show was particularly difficult, with a heavy costume and technically demanding fast work. An injury to another dancer meant that he had to do all the performances without any cover. Then someone else was injured and he had to learn their new part in another work from video, at the same time as rehearsing for a triple bill. His leg started aching and became steadily worse. Then in a matinee performance he felt his leg 'go'. The company physiotherapist suspected a stress fracture. However, he had to go on for the evening show because there was no cover. This aggravated the injury and he had to be off work for six months.

Overuse injuries have a more subtle onset than traumatic injuries. The first sign is pain after activity. There is usually a gradual increase of pain associated with a particular, usually repetitive, activity. Then there is pain during activity.

These conditions are more difficult for the athlete or dancer, coach and sports medicine professional to accept, recognise and diagnose because they may be confused with diseases or inflammatory conditions with similar pain patterns. The dancer, teacher or company may be reluctant to recognise overuse injury and inclined to 'work through' the pain because of the career or performance implications. The advantage of homoeopathic treatment in such conditions is that regardless of the pathological source of the symptoms such as pain, swelling, heat, restlessness and irritability, a remedy can often be prescribed to remove the general effect on the individual and cure the condition more swiftly.

You may wish to refer the patient for a medical assessment for your own peace of mind, but you will find, with experience, that certain homoeopathic remedies seem to fit certain common conditions. It may also be appropriate to refer the patient to a professional homoeopath for treatment.

Warm Up

As prevention is always better than cure I must take this opportunity to stress the importance of warming up before, and warming down after, all physical exercise and activity. As a mountaineer and rock climber I am often surprised at the many climbers who set off on a route without warming up before climbing. They then expect their ligaments and tendons to stretch, their joints to be mobile and their muscles strong without the least preparation. Golfing friends laugh at the idea of warming up before playing, and then consult me about their aching backs and shoulders. I often observe people come into the conditioning room and start using weights with only the most minimal attempt at warm up.

Louis Galli, *Dance Magazine*, 1994, found that dancers who warmed up before every performance were injured 70% less often than those who did not.

Every exercise session should start with a gradual warm up and end with a warm down, followed by a shower or bath. The warm up, lasting a minimum of 15 minutes, and ideally 30 minutes, should consist of four parts:

1) Stretching session: passive stretching of the main muscle groups.
2) Mobilising: ballistic bending exercises for the joints.
3) Cardiovascular warmers: five to ten sets of 30 seconds each of harder exercises designed to increase the pulse rate.
4) Quiet skills practice: mental rehearsal and preparation for the event or exercise.

Care should also be taken not to cool down between warm up and competition, main activity or performance.

Warm Down

Warm down with more gentle stretching, relaxation routines, meditation, reflection on the performance and gentle positive reinforcing repetitions of exercises until the mind and body are at rest and recovered.

The Highly-Trained Performer

Development of overuse conditions in highly-trained, fit and healthy performers can be ascribed to two main causes; performance stress and altered internal state. The altered internal state can often be produced by the stress of long term or intense performance. In these days when the demands on athletes or dancers are becoming extreme, the occurrences of injuries one sees and reads of are becoming more frequent, and more serious. Anything that helps an athlete or dancer cope with these demands must be welcome.

Performance Stress

Longer and longer seasons, overseas tours, increasingly important matches and the need for professional athletes to perform, perform and perform again at top levels all produce and increase mental and emotional stress in the individual as well as the obvious physical stress. This prolonged stress inevitably leads to injury and deteriorating performance. The susceptibility to injury, infection and illness caused by the accumulation of wear, tear and stress is the biggest risk the athlete faces. His judgement will suffer and he is likely to suffer more frequent injuries.

'The wide open vistas of the North American landscape seem to embrace the six dancers and goad them on to even greater endeavour. And even greater energy, too. For this must be one of the most taxing ballets these dancers have ever had to face, a half hour of relentless, panting physical exertion that pushed even the Amazonian Darcey Bussell to the brink of exhaustion on opening night.' (*The Times*, May 2, 1997).

Dancers suffer more from the effects of long-term mental and emotional stress than any other physical performers, and from an early age have to learn to cope with the sometimes excessive demands of choreography, the anxiety of performance and stage fright, depression, performance related stress and lack of self esteem. None of this is helped by the average dancer and student's economic stress and poverty.

Warning Signs

There are warning signals for overuse injuries. When they become more frequent, and when the performer becomes 'injury prone', he or she needs rest. These early signals are listed overleaf.

WARNING SIGNALS FOR OVERUSE INJURY

Physical	*Mental*	*General*
1) Stiffness and pain during exercise or normal activity.	Poor concentration.	Lacks energy.
2) Sense of low-grade fever or infection.	Agitation.	Easy fatigue.
3) Frequent colds.	Feels diffuse, detached and remote.	Poor performance.
4) Cold sores and/or mouth ulcers.	Increased irritability.	Loss of co-ordination.
5) Frequent minor injury.	Depression.	Increased resting pulse and respiration rate.
6) Cuts, bruises, abrasions.	Anxiety.	Increased sweating. Cold sweats.
7) Swelling, inflammation.	Fastidious.	Sleep problems, increased dreaming, early waking.
8) Sprains and strains.	Breaks routine.	Increased sensitivity to weather conditions.
9) Stress and other fractures.	Jealousy, paranoia, tantrums.	Dehydration.
10) Pain following activity.	Increased anxiety in anticipation of performance. 'Stage fright.' Lowered self-esteem.	

Short-Term, High-Stress Events

Short-term protracted competitions, tournaments or performances, where an athlete or dancer has to perform at top level four or five times within a short period of time, involve much physical and mental stress. In tournaments or performances where the sport involves body contact or the possibility of strenuous violent activity the build up of stress increases in direct proportion to the length of the tournament. Warming up and down and relaxation between performances is important. There are also homoeopathic remedies that will help. When considering these it is important to recognise the changes that may occur in the performer as the result of stress and to prescribe according to those changes. Some useful remedies are discussed below and in Chapter 11.

Preparation

Preparation for intense competition and an increased level of performance is obviously essential, and most performers, coaches and managers recognise this need. Sometimes athletes or dancers are called on to compete at a higher level than normal or in an unaccustomed position, event or choreography.

Support the athlete or dancer in this eventuality with Arnica, and be conscious of the potential effects of the stress in causing minor ailments.

The coach, manager or professional carer should recognise the mental and physical changes in athletes or dancers during long tournaments or tours and as an intense and demanding season progresses. Minor injuries can build up gradually into serious debilitating conditions that undermine an athlete or dancer's performance. It would be best to treat those minor injuries early and effectively to prevent the accumulation. The mental and general changes are often the first to appear, but may be the last to be noticed.

Arnica

Participants in long and intense tournaments would benefit from a daily dose of Arnica 30c for the duration of the tournament. This would help their recovery after each event or match. It will also help them to recover from minor knocks and bruises and their accumulated effects.

The Effects of Long-Term Activity

We must recognise the effects of intensive and protracted competition or performance on athletes and dancers, and how their positive attributes and mental approach may become negative. This change can lead to injury.

Anxiety and Fatigue

For example, you have an athlete or dancer in your care who is normally anxious before an event. He is capable of performing well

71

with that level of anxiety, and the anxiety helps his performance. You notice during the later stages of a long competition that his anxiety develops into a recognisable fear of failure. He begins to say that he would prefer not to play in case he may lose, and suffers a loss of incentive to go on. He may develop aching, tired legs. His head and legs feel heavy. He sleeps, but seems unrefreshed. Perhaps he cannot sleep, despite being very tired and sleepy. He simply wants to rest and to be kept cool. This person may first approach you because of his leg symptoms.

Picric Acid
An athlete or dancer with these symptoms would benefit from one tablet of Picric Acid 200c. This remedy will help him to overcome the effects of prolonged anxiety.

Recognising the Condition

Sports men and women tend to be very conscious of their bodies and physical condition. They are unlikely to start telling you about their mental and emotional state. It is the role of the skilled sports medicine professional, coach, manager or fellow athlete or dancer to be able to recognise changes that occur in the person who needs help. At this level help would best be obtained from a professionally qualified homoeopath, but if you have the experience and ability to assess a person's needs there can be little harm in trying an indicated remedy for one or two doses.

Recognising Changes

It is important to recognise the change from a determined, active, stimulating performer to one whose attitude has altered so that the positive attributes have become negative. It is a question of degree, and control. A certain level of anxiety, nervousness, excitability and stress is essential for any good performer at sport, dance or any other physical activity. The better the performer or athlete, the higher level of stress they can utilise and control. The stress itself becomes a stimulant to improved performance.

The same anxiety, excitability and nervousness can become pathological when they continue for longer than the athlete or dancer's constitution can respond positively to. They then run out of control. The constitution responds in a protective way. They become susceptible to injuries which develop gradually in response to overuse. An underlying weakness in the body predisposes it to break down under stressed conditions in even the best trained and prepared person if the intensity or length of competition, season, or classes demands too much of them.

Acute trauma can be the result of more subtle causes, and the responsible coach, manager or trainer must be aware of this. In the end, of course, it is the dancer, athlete or performer who must be in touch with his or her 'body/mind' and its state of health. The onset of acute injuries, and their frequency, deserve to be treated as signals for the need to examine one's overall level of conditioning, training and emotional and mental attitude to performance.

Although it is tempting to read your own character into the above table, and many of the above attributes are fundamental to quality performance, remember that it is when these characteristics become overemphasised to a debilitating level that they become symptoms of potential overuse injury. When that happens it is time to take a rest, mentally, emotionally and physically, and to restore the energies that may have become depleted. Relaxation, meditation, a change of schedule and homoeopathy can all help.

Remedies for Stress

Because most stress symptoms manifest themselves as mental and emotional states which have become exaggerated beyond the control of the individual it may be better to consult a professional homoeopath for the correct prescription.

Many of the conditions described below are a natural part of the performer's psyche. It is when they become uncontrollable and debilitating, or adversely affect the athlete or dancer's performance that they may be regarded as requiring treatment.

Here are a few remedies which I have found useful in dealing with cumulative stress. Choose the remedy that seems closer to the person's symptom picture, then give one tablet daily for three days in the 200c potency.

Arsenicum Album
Oversensitive, anxious, and fault-finding after prolonged strenuous exertion. Very fastidious about appearance and clothes, and inclined to seek many opinions about injury or health. Likes to be kept very warm and wrapped up. May be suspicious and irritable when tired. Restless legs when tired. Restless generally, and in sleep, which may be disturbed. Intense thirst for little sips of water. Cannot bear the sight or smell of food. Burning diarrhoea. Complete exhaustion.

Bryonia

Exceedingly irritable. Apprehension and dread of the future. May become very ugly in behaviour. Wants to go home. Physically very reluctant to move at all because even the slightest movement is painful. Wants to lie quietly without even speaking. Pain does not improve with continued movement. Any exertion makes it worse. Joints are red, swollen and hot. Excessive thirst.

Cocculus

For sleeplessness after extreme physical and mental exhaustion. 'Too tired to sleep.' Anxious, confused, introspective, and forgetful. Time passes too quickly. Profound sadness, for example at the end of a demanding dance project or sports tour, especially one that required much travelling. Trembling and pain in the limbs.

Gelsemium

Flu that comes on suddenly after extremely demanding exercise or exertion. Almost paralysing exhaustion. Cold symptoms that take several days to develop, and are slow to come on. Sneezing, red face, heavy eyelids, cold limbs, aching in all joints, headache and drowsiness. Develops flu-like symptoms. Weakness and soreness in muscles, shivering, heavy eyes, coldness in back. Legs give out.

Kali Carbonicum

Catches colds easily after exhausting exertion. Develops a cough with wheezing and chest pain. Angry, irritable, quarrelsome and anxious. Needs company and dislikes being alone, but also quarrels with companions. Dislikes being touched. Weakness, legs give out, back pains, sciatica. Amenorrhea in dancers and athletes.

Natrum Muriaticum

Remote and unapproachable, angrily rejects sympathy or caring. Feels very weak on waking from sleep. Keeps things very much to herself.

Nux Vomica

Normally a quick, active, nervous, successful, hard-working person; becomes very irritable, impatient, angry and violent when exhausted. Restless. Prone to cramp in calves and soles of feet. Legs become weak and stiff from overexertion.

Picric Acid (see pages 71–2)

74

Sudden Increase of Activity

There can be few physical performers or participants in physical activity who have not experienced the results of indulging in unaccustomed physical activity. From the gardener after his spring digging, the walker who takes on a longer, harder route than usual, to the footballer after his or her first early season training session and the dancer returning after injury or rest, we have all felt stiffness the following morning. Similarly, a sudden change in training routine, such as increasing running mileage from twenty to sixty miles a week, or doubling weight training schedules, even training every day after only training three times a week, can make your body respond by showing signs of overwork.

A change of footwear, training, practice or performing surface can have similar results.

A too-early return to training or playing after illness or injury can also produce signs of overuse in the affected parts or a recurrence of the condition. It is important to make a full functional recovery after a layoff, and to return to dancing, training or playing gradually, doing a little at a time. Overuse can affect the other limb as the athlete or dancer favours the injured one. Warming up and warming down are even more important for athletes or dancers returning to sport or training after a rest.

Overexertion

Well-trained, fitter individuals, with highly vascularised muscle tissue will suffer more bleeding subsequent to muscle injury. Many of the effects of overexertion are similar to those of the shock following trauma. Older performers are likely to suffer more intramuscular bleeding, inflammation and swelling after muscle injury. They may suffer similar effects after unusual strenuous activity, during and after long term exercise, and in other circumstances where overuse injuries may occur.

Both groups are likely to suffer the effects of overexertion. Immediate administration of Arnica to both groups will make recovery swifter and more effective. I often advise people to take one Arnica before a programmed strenuous training session.

In some cases, where the sports person or dancer consults a practitioner some time after an injury, it could be beneficial to give them one Arnica 200c to start their treatment.

Pain as a Signal

Although stiffness after a training session may be expected after a lay-off, continuing stiffness resulting from excessive training can lead to further injuries. Playing or exercising 'through' an injury or pain can only do further harm to the part. If any movement or activity is painful this must be regarded as a sign that the activity or movement must be stopped. After the necessary first treatment an accurate diagnosis must be the first priority. A programme of stretching, strengthening and functional rehabilitation supervised by a chartered physiotherapist should follow every injury in preparation for restarting training or playing. The correct homoeopathic remedy will also help.

CASE 13

An estate agent and recreational runner normally ran fifteen miles a week at a relaxed pace. An osteopath colleague had referred him because he had told her about his headaches and dizzy feeling. He had consulted her about unexplained soreness in both knees. There was stiffness in both legs, and cracking in both knees when he moved them, cramp in his calves and pain in his right forearm.

I noticed he was restless, and stretched his legs frequently. He is an impatient hard worker, whose wife describes him as a 'workaholic'. He had become more irritable since his knees had started hurting. He never eats breakfast and likes to get the morning over quickly. The dizziness was worse mid-morning, when he also felt hungry. He normally enjoyed coffee and a glass or two of wine, but recently found that coffee made him more irritable, and had started having headaches in the morning after a few glasses of wine the evening before. The problems arose after his recent decision to train with a younger, fitter runner, and an increase to twenty-five miles a week at a faster pace than before.

Comment

Nux Vomica was the remedy that best fitted the above symptoms, and he took two doses of the 200c potency for three days. I advised him to train with his new partner only once a week at first, and to build up his distance and speed gradually. One week later he was running gently, and after six weeks had built up his schedules to those he was enjoying before his injuries stopped him.

The symptoms that led to the prescription of Nux Vomica were:

1) Impatience, irritability and anger.
2) Works too hard.
3) Ailments from overexertion.
4) Worse early morning.
5) Desires wine and coffee, which may disagree.
6) Restlessness.
7) Vertigo on empty stomach.
8) Cracking in knees, stiffness of legs.

You may notice that I decided on the prescription more from the mental and general symptoms than from his stiff and cracking knees.

Remedies for Overexertion

Arnica
Taken before a hard training session, one Arnica 6c will prevent the muscle stiffness from usually strenuous activity. Taken after an un-accustomed hard session or performance, it will have the same effect. It will prevent the bruising that accompanies overexertion.
Dosage: One Arnica 6c, before a training session, and one following if necessary.

Arsenicum Album
Becomes oversensitive, anxious and fault-finding after prolonged strenuous exertion. Very fastidious about appearance and clothes, and inclined to seek many opinions about injury or health. Likes to be kept very warm and wrapped up. May be suspicious and irritable when tired. Restless legs when tired. Restless generally, and in sleep, which may be disturbed.
Dosage: One Arsenicum Album 200c. There should be no need to repeat the remedy if the state improves after one dose. Give one more if it does not improve after two or three days.

Bryonia
Very reluctant to move at all. Wants to lie quietly without even speak-ing. Every movement, even the slightest, is painful. Pain does not improve with continued movement. Any exertion makes it worse. Wants to go home. May become very irritable and ugly in behaviour. Joints red, swollen and hot.
Dosage: One Bryonia 6c will help him to get moving.

Cocculus

For sleeplessness after extreme physical and mental exhaustion. Describes herself as 'too tired to sleep.'

Dosage: One Cocculus 30c or 200c. Only one dose of the 200c should be given.

Gelsemium

Develops flu-like symptoms after extremely demanding exercise or exertion. Weakness and soreness in muscles, shivering, heavy eyes, coldness in back, drowsiness, disinclined towards further exertion.

Dosage: One Gelsemium 6c.

Natrum Muriaticum

Becomes remote and unapproachable, and certainly does not want sympathy or caring. Feels very weak on waking from sleep.

Dosage: One Natrum Muriaticum 6c.

Nux Vomica

Normally quick, active, nervous, successful, hard-working; becomes very irritable, impatient, angry and violent when exhausted. Restless. Prone to cramp in the calves and soles of feet. Legs become weak and stiff from overexertion.

Dosage: One Nux Vomica 6c.

Rhus Toxicodendron

Taken after a hard training session or performance, Rhus Tox. will eradicate the bruised and painful stiffness that could follow. It will ensure a good night's sleep when normally one would be restless and unable to find comfortable position. First motion is painful but the pain and stiffness ease with continued movement. Rhus Tox. is very useful after early season training.

Dosage: One Rhus Toxicodendron 6c following a training session, if necessary.

Ruta

Intense painful weariness after exertion. Restlessness with sore aching pains felt mainly in the ligaments and tendons or deep in the bones. Walking up and down steps is especially painful. Sleep difficult because the longer the person lies in one position the worse he feels.

Dosage: One Ruta 6c following a training session if necessary.

Chapter 8

Local Treatment for Specific Injuries

The following sections give suggestions or remedies for specific and local injuries and conditions. It has often been my experience that the person's constitutional remedy heals more effectively than the specific remedy. However, the specific remedy will often serve the practitioner of other therapies who wants to choose a remedy to relieve a patient's immediate symptoms and promote recovery. This chapter suggests remedies according to locations of injuries, but also includes supporting symptoms for selected remedies.

Although the conditions and injuries may not be described as specifically applying to dancers, it is important to realise that the process of choosing a remedy is the same for injuries whatever the activity. A dancer with sesamoiditis could find the condition as much relieved by Ledum as a runner would.

Although I generally recommend the 30c potency for injuries because I have found it to be most effective, do not hesitate to use the 6c potency if it is the only one available from the pharmacy or health food shop. In all cases, if the first chosen remedy does not seem to have any effect after five or six doses, it should be replaced with another remedy.

THE FOOT

The foot is a sensitive extremity. Reflexologists believe that every organ and system in the human body has a corresponding area in the foot. By manipulating the correct area a skilled reflexologist may be able to treat any disease or condition. Foot massage is certainly useful for relaxing or stimulating the whole body and the whole person. Injuries to the foot are reflected throughout the person.

The normal foot is resilient and strong, flexible and rigid, and is required to be stable, shock absorbing and responsive. It is capable of absorbing huge forces and springing back into shape immediately. It is capable of launching a person into the air, calculating the amount of absorption necessary for his return to land and preparing for the next launch in any direction chosen.

Most sports involve some sort of walking, running, or jumping, and dance involves the feet in every element of the art. A dancer's foot may need to absorb forces two or three times more than his body weight, and this may be repeated thousands of times during a performance. A runner's foot has similar stress. The high incidence of conditions affecting the feet in sports and dance, the latter especially, is a reflection of the fact that the foot is normally the performer's first contact with the ground.

It is no wonder that foot injuries can be among the most painful and debilitating. Foot pain can be very depressing, and may cause nausea, headaches and general malaise. Foot injuries account for 6% of injuries seen in the Peter Wilson Sports Injuries Clinic (Lachman and Jenner). They account for more than 20% of injuries to dancers (Brinson and Dick).

Bony Injuries

The foot contains twenty-six bones. Some are relatively long, others are tiny and yet others thick and square. They form three arches which help to give the foot its springiness. Two tiny extra bones are found beneath the ball of the big toe. These are called sesamoids, and can cause a problem when the surrounding area becomes inflamed.

Phosphorus

Phosphorus is a specific remedy for inflammation under the ball of the big toe. There is burning pain and numbness, and the person totters when walking.
Dosage: One Phosphorus 30c, daily for three days.

Sesamoiditis

This may be suspected when there is tenderness and some loose swelling in the pad behind the big toe or hallux. I have found Ledum to be effective for this condition, especially when the person avoids moving the joint and is worse at night. An orthotic pad prescribed by a podiatrist will help to relieve the condition.
Dosage: One Ledum 30c, daily for three days.

Calcaneum Spur

A calcaneum or heel spur is a small bony outgrowth on the front part of the heel. It may make walking and running painful. If a calcaneum spur develops and causes problems, in addition to appropriate heel pads to redistribute the weight on the heel, there are three remedies that may help:

Calcarea Fluorica
Calc. Fluor. is recommended for all indurations and swellings around tendons, and can arrest the development of bony growths. It may also reduce exostoses.
Dosage: One Calc. Fluor. 30c, daily for three days.

Hecla Lava
This remedy has been known to reduce bony spurs and other exostoses.
Dosage: One Hecla 30c, daily for two weeks.

Silica
Bruised, throbbing pain in the heel which prevents walking, nails are rough, brittle, blue or black. Tends to have weak ankles and feet. Cramp in soles of feet. Bad smelling foot sweat. Wants to be kept warm, and cannot bear cold, touch or pressure. Worse at night. May have lost confidence.
Dosage: One Silica 30c three time daily until relief is felt, or for three days. But first read the warning on page 264.

Bruised Heel

This can be caused by repeated heavy landing on the heel, commonly from jumping, but also from long walks or runs on hard surfaces. The heel feels sore when pressure is applied, such as when walking or standing.

Arnica
One Arnica 6c, immediately the pain is felt, or to prevent ill effects following a long walk or run.

Badiaga
This remedy will relieve the pain in the heel when the slightest pressure hurts, and touch is unbearable. The pain may be associated with skin soreness.
Dosage: One Badiaga 6c, as necessary for the pain, but do not repeat for more than three days in succession.

CASE 14

A rock climber jumped down a few feet from a climb and landed on his heel. The pain was excruciating and shocking. He felt nauseous, and wanted to be left alone and quiet. He refused to remove his boot because he feared it would hurt. He said, 'I'm fine, I'm OK. Don't worry, I'll just go home.' But he could only walk with great difficulty, and certainly did not want to go to a hospital.

I was climbing nearby and gave him Arnica 30c. Within minutes he was feeling less shocked and nauseous, agreed to have his boot taken off, and to be driven to hospital where he was found to have suffered a fracture to his calcaneum.

Fractures and Dislocations

Fractures and dislocations of the toes and metatarsals, and conditions such as calcaneal apophysitis and osteochondritis of the head of metatarsals should be dealt with homoeopathically according to the symptoms. The correct remedy in combination with suitable and appropriate physical therapy will almost certainly help healing. See the section below on stress fractures and foot pain to help you choose the best remedy.

Stress Fractures of the Metatarsals

Stress fractures are partial or complete fractures of bone, often called fatigue fractures since they are caused by repetitive strain during sub-maximal activity. They result from the inability of the bone to react favourably to the stress imposed. The lower limbs tend to be the most common sites for stress fractures, and they tend to be more frequent in runners than in all the other sports put together. The most frequent stress fracture suffered by runners and dancers tend to be in the tibia, but the metatarsals come second.

Risk Factors

The risk of stress fractures seems to increase with age, especially in older women. They commonly appear after a change in activity and an increase in running mileage and intensity. Other risk factors seem to be:

- If training is resumed at the same level after a layoff.
- Beginners overtraining from misguided enthusiasm.
- Excessive running on hard surfaces and on cambered roads.
- Intensive dance class on hard surfaces.

- Sedentary, overweight and unfit people entering a training programme.
- Menopausal women, women with irregular menstrual cycles, and girls entering dance and training programmes at the onset of menstruation.
- A high arch in the foot, excessive pronation and supination of the foot, a bunion on the big toe and a longer second toe will all impose abnormal stresses on the bones of the foot and leg.

The best advice for avoiding stress fractures is to approach training in a sensible and gradual way, and for the athlete, coach and teacher to be aware of the risks involved.

Newer running shoes in good condition seem to produce fewer fractures.

The Risk to Dancers and Gymnasts

Dancers themselves judge their self-worth and self-esteem from their ability to keep going, and believe that even one day's rest can lead to loss of skill. They tend to ignore the early warning signs of injury, try to treat themselves and avoid referring to a specialist. Most injuries to dancers occur in rehearsal, and about 20% of injuries occur to the lower leg. Unsuitable floors could be an important factor in causing overuse and stress fractures among dancers (Brinson and Dick).

Gymnasts have been found to suffer similar problems to those described for dancers.

Pain During Exercise

The most significant symptom of stress fracture is the presence of pain during exercise. The injury is first noticed as an area of tenderness around the bone. Pain is felt during class training or performance but not at rest. It increases in intensity with continued training. The pain may develop gradually or appear suddenly. Later it persists after exercise has ceased, and local tenderness and swelling may be evident.

Rest

Rest is the most important component of treatment for all stress fractures, and that rest must be total. In other conditions I have recommended that the athlete should continue to exercise. When one has suffered a stress fracture the temptation to 'try out' the injury is great. Training should not be resumed until the athlete or dancer has been free of pain for a minimum of ten days, and when training restarts it must stop again if pain recurs.

Return to Activity

The return to activity must be gradual, progressive and – through varied exercises – well monitored and careful, especially for dance and running. Non-weight bearing exercise such as swimming or cycling should be used to maintain cardiovascular and pulmonary fitness.

Homoeopathic Treatment for Stress Fractures

Homoeopathic treatment for stress fractures should be given in three stages:

Phase 1:

Arnica

Arnica should be given immediately the pain is felt, and rest from high impact activity is essential, if the pain is sore and there is bruising, touch is painful and the person insists he is well enough to continue per-forming.

Dosage: One Arnica 30c, repeated hourly for three or four doses.

Phase 2:

Bryonia

If any movement is painful. The pain increases as activity continues, and decreases with rest. Pressing or firm bandaging the area eases the pain.

Dosage: Bryonia 30c three times a day can make movement and weight-bearing easier. This should be continued as necessary until the pain begins to ease, but not longer than a week.

Rhus Toxicodendron

If the pain is typically worse for first movement, better with continued movement. It is difficult to find a comfortable position to rest and the person moves the foot constantly. Pain is worse at night.

Dosage: Rhus Tox. 30c, one tablet twice a day for three days, or until the pain eases.

Rhododendron

Rhododendron has a bruised, drawing and tearing pain in the bone. The feet feel cold, even in a warm room and in bed. There is weakness after even slight exertion, and the person is sensitive to windy, stormy weather. Heat reduces the discomfort.

Dosage: Rhododendron 30c, three times a day for three days, or until the pain eases.

Phase 3:

Symphytum

One tablet of Symphytum 6c, three times daily for two weeks will help the bones to heal. Then stop the remedy for a week and start again for another two weeks.

See also below for general foot pain remedies.

Hallux Rigidus and Osteochondritis

Stiffness of the big toe joint is a gradual process, often the result of earlier injury to the big toe and its joint with the head of the metatarsal during growth in adolescence. The pain is worse during forceful bending such as when sprinting or lunging. Osteochondritis is inflammation of the big toe joint following the deterioration of the bone ends as the result of childhood or adolescent trauma to the toe. Both of these conditions produce pain and tenderness between the toe and the head of the metatarsal.

Bryonia

In hallux rigidus the pain is felt with the least movement, especially dorsiflexion. Bryonia will help to make movement and walking less painful. It may be taken orally for as long as necessary to relieve the pain and this may eliminate the necessity for surgery.

Dosage: One Bryonia 30c, as necessary until the pain eases, but not longer than a week.

Ledum Palustre

In osteochondritis when pain is felt behind the toes and movement is not only painful but actually makes the pain worse. Cold applications ease the pain and warmth makes it worse. There may also be swelling and tenderness

Dosage: One Ledum 30c, until the pain ceases, but not longer than a week.

Gradually-Developing Foot Pain

Gradually-developing foot pain can be caused by an inflammatory joint condition such as gout or ankylosing spondylitis, or it could be referred pain from a back problem. Although these conditions can be treated successfully with homoeopathic medicine, one should refer the patient for a diagnosis by a doctor and treatment by a qualified homoeopath.

Ligament Injuries and Conditions

Ligaments bind the foot bones together and act as springs, giving the foot resilience and strength. The two ligaments most likely to cause trouble are the plantar fascia and the spring ligament.

Any of the many ligaments in the foot may be strained by trauma or overuse. If a sudden tearing pain is felt Arnica should be taken as soon as possible. Once ligament damage is suspected Ruta 30c should be taken three times a day until an improvement is felt, but for no longer than a week.

Plantar Fasciitis and Tears

Inflammation of the plantar fascia may occur in sports which involve repeated jumping, or forced dorsiflexion of the foot, such as in long uphill walks. Wearing shoes with lower than usual heels, or running and walking in thin soled shoes or bare feet may also cause this condition. It is the most common cause of heel pain in runners and is a common cause of foot pain in dancers.

If the plantar fascia partly detaches from the calcaneum it can cause local pain and tenderness. The tear may be caused by jumping, stepping down or is worse when walking, standing or an unexpected dorsiflexion of the foot such as partially stepping on a stone or kerb.

This condition may take a long time to heal. The remedies listed under the 'Foot Pain in General' section on page 91 may help. The person will almost certainly need a dose of Arnica if there has been trauma.

The pain may be felt on the bottom of the foot near the heel. Prolonged and repeated tension of the fascia, which extends from the calcaneum to the heads of the metatarsals, causes bleeding. A sudden increase in activity or a change of activity can be the cause of this injury. Typically the heel hurts when standing after a period of rest, and eases up after repeated or continued movement. Mechanical treatment by taping, and the provision of soft orthotics can play an important part in recovery. Healing may take up to four weeks.

Arnica
Dosage: One Arnica 6c or 30c. Two or three doses if there was trauma following unaccustomed or increased exercise or activity, or when the pain is first felt.

Graphites
If there is burning pain when in bed.
Dosage: One Graphites 30c.

Rhododendron
Rhododendron has a bruised, drawing and tearing pain in the heel. The feet feel cold, even in a warm room and in bed. There is weakness after even slight exertion, and the person is sensitive to windy, stormy weather. Heat reduces the discomfort.
Dosage: One Rhododendron 30c, three times a day for not longer than a week, or until the pain eases.

Rhus Toxicodendron
As if stepping on a stone. If the pain is typically worse for first movement, better with continued movement. It is difficult to find a comfortable position to rest and the person moves the foot constantly. Pain is worse at night.
Dosage: Rhus Tox. 30c, one tablet twice a day for a few days until the pain eases, but not longer than a week.

Ruta
Ruta has a special affinity with ligaments and tendons, and should be used when you suspect strain, damage or inflammation in the ligaments or tendons of the foot. It will often be effective when the foot pain is the result of overuse, and when there is pain from the slightest physical exertion. Bruised, sore and aching pain is felt near the heel.
Dosage: One Ruta 30c, daily for up to a week. Stop when relief is felt.

Zinc
The pain is very exhausting.
Dosage: One Zinc 30c.

Spring Ligament Strain

This ligament may also be strained by a change in normal activity or trauma. Treatment is similar to that for plantar fasciitis according to the symptoms. (See also 'Foot Pain in General', page 91.)

Heel Pain – Plantar Fascia Tear

A plantar fascia tear may be caused by a sudden exertion, stepping down, jumping or dorsiflexion of the foot when the agonistic and antagonistic muscles are not acting. The condition is noticed by a sudden tearing pain near the middle of the arch during exercise. The victim is usually middle-aged or elderly, and there may be some danger of an arch collapse if the injury is not treated. This painful and debilitating condition is often very slow to heal, and may prevent participation or performance for more than six weeks while the ligament heals. A further complication may arise if a bony spur grows from the calcaneum, causing further pain, and complications further up the locomotor framework.

The injury requires continued RICE (Rest, Ice, Compression and Elevation).

Contrast baths may also help healing by stimulating circulation. This treatment is simple to carry out at home using two buckets or bowls. One is filled with iced water, and the other with water as hot as can be borne without discomfort. The foot is dipped into one bowl and kept there for a few seconds. Then the foot is taken out, dried, and put in the other bowl. The sequence may be repeated for ten minutes or so, or until the skin begins to flush.

Angustura Vera
Sudden tearing pain in foot, cannot put it down. Limps badly. Much better from cold applications, especially cold hands, and worse during rest. Constant thirst.
Dosage: One Angustura 30c, every hour during pain, for up to six doses.

Arnica
Dosage: One Arnica 6c or 30c immediately and repeat for six one-hourly doses.

Kali Carbonicum

Tearing pain in the sole caused by a sudden, unguarded movement. Very sensitive to touch. Does not like cold. Pain is worse in the middle of the night, 2 to 3 a.m., and the person is anxious and quarrelsome.
Dosage: One Kali Carb. 30c, three times daily for three days.

Symphytum

Dosage: One Symphytum 30c, taken every day for two weeks will promote healing.

Physiotherapy, using ultrasound and friction should be provided. NSAIDs should not be necessary if Arnica and Symphytum, or the other indicated remedies as described for the foot, are used. Note that Symphytum may be given at the same time as another indicated remedy because it acts as a tissue repair agent. (See also 'Fractures', page 100.)

Calcaneal Apophysitis (Sever's Disease)

Apophysitis of the calcaneum, inflammatory pain in the heel, is commonly caused by repetitive jarring on hard surfaces, which can occur in young dancers and very active children who run and jump on hard floors, for example in practising gymnastics. Pain is felt down the sides of the heel, and any pressure on the heel hurts.

Arnica

Arnica should be taken as soon as the discomfort and pain arise. Rest and non-jarring exercise are essential for recovery.
Dosage: One Arnica 30c, as necessary.

Badiaga

This remedy will relieve the pain from pressure if even the slightest pressure hurts and the part cannot be touched.
Dosage: One Badiaga 30c, as necessary for the pain, for not more than three days.

Conium Maculatum

For shooting pains in the heel, with a feeling that there is a lump or stone under the heel and that the bone would push out. The person may stagger when walking. This remedy is often indicated for older people.
Dosage: One Conium 30c, as necessary for the pain, for three days.

Pulsatilla

The young athlete or dancer experiences the worst pain down the sides of the heel when beginning to walk, and in the evening. Likely to forget the pain as soon as the mind is taken by another interest. May be weepy.

Dosage: One Pulsatilla 30c, three times a day for seven days.

Rhododendron

Rhododendron has a bruised, drawing and tearing pain in the heel. The feet feel cold, even in a warm room and in bed. The pain, when walking, may be felt more in the Achilles tendon. There is weakness after even slight exertion, and the person is sensitive to windy, stormy weather. Heat reduces the discomfort.

Dosage: One Rhododendron 30c, three times a day for not more than a week, or until the pain eases.

Symphytum

See page 89 above.

Tenosynovitis of Dorsiflexor Tendons

If the maintaining cause of a condition can be identified, it should be removed. If the tenosynovitis is caused by overtightening shoelaces, the laces should be loosened or padding provided. Ruta ointment or cream will help to ease pain and reduce inflammation.

Black Toenail (Subungual Haematoma)

The toenail of the big toe is particularly susceptible to bruising from walking or running downhill for long periods, wearing shoes that are too short or narrow for dance or running, or from a blow to the toe. The injury is very painful at first because of bleeding into the restricted space under the nail. If the pressure is not relieved the pain becomes unbearable and throbbing in nature, and the nail eventually becomes detached from the toe.

The best method of relieving pressure is trephining. Heat a paper clip and burn a hole in the nail. This may seem drastic but it is actually painless. Better still, one could prevent the swelling by limiting the extravasation with a dose or two of Arnica as soon as the condition becomes obvious.

Remedies for the condition of black toenail are as follows.

Arnica
As soon as the toe begins to feel bruised, Arnica will prevent bleeding under the nail and swelling. Use immediately if the swelling, pain and bruising is because of a blow to the toe.
Dosage: Just one tablet of the 30c potency should be enough.

Arsenicum Album
This remedy is specific for discoloured toenails when they have gone black. It is more painful after midnight, the person cannot bear cold in any form, is very restless and becomes very weak, even from a sore toe. In other words, the Arsenicum patient suffers out of proportion to the seriousness of his condition.
Dosage: One Arsenicum 30c, three times in one day.

Hypericum
If the pain becomes unbearable and shoots into the foot or leg after bleeding under the nail.
Dosage: One Hypericum 30, as required for the pain.

Silica
Bruised, throbbing pain in toe. Pain prevents walking, nails are rough, brittle, blue or black. Noticeably bad-smelling foot sweat. Wants to be kept warm and cannot bear cold, touch or pressure. Worse at night. May have lost confidence.
Dosage: One Silica 200c. (But first note the warning on page 264.)

Foot Pain in General
The remedies suggested below will be found effective for all foot pain as indicated by the symptoms, including plantar fasciitis, metatarsalgia, sesamoiditis, intrinsic muscle strain, and spring ligament strain.

Whatever the anatomical or mechanical cause, and regardless of the diagnosis, you can prescribe for foot pain according to the homoeopathic symptoms. You may use several remedies successfully in association with physiotherapy or osteopathy and RICE if you take care to match the symptoms to the remedy. Some of the most likely remedies are listed overleaf.

Arnica

If the pain started from a fall, blow or sudden twisting, stretching, dorsiflexion or plantar flexion, or if the injury was of a traumatic nature of any sort then the first remedy must be Arnica 30c. It is especially required if there is bruising or the chance of bruising. The patient does not want treatment, says he is 'fine' when he obviously is not, and avoids coming close to people because he fears that if they touch him the pain will increase. He avoids putting his foot on the ground for the same reason. He may feel bruised all over, not only in the foot, and may feel weak in his knees.

Dosage: One Arnica 30c, one or two doses.

Arsenicum Album

Soreness and burning in the ball of the toe when walking (sesamoiditis), the feet feel weak and numb, soles may feel numb. Wants heat treatment. Very restless, cannot sit in one place and moves from chair to chair. Cannot bear cold in any form, may shiver, and needs to be kept warmly dressed or wrapped up. May refuse ice treatment however well indicated. Very fastidious about personal appearance, details of performance, treatment. May consult several doctors or practitioners, but is also very careful with money. May even seem stingy.

Dosage: One Arsenicum 30c, once daily until the pain is relieved, or for three days.

Aurum Metallicum

Where there is a bruised pain in the soles of the feet and they are hot at night. The pain may also be sharp and boring, and may be felt deep in the foot. The Aurum patient may be depressed and brooding about the injury, and can get angry quickly. Likes music, and moonlight.

Dosage: One Aurum 30c, twice a day for three days.

Bryonia

The pain in the feet is like pins and needles, and they are swollen and hot. The soles are painful as soon as they touch the ground, but are better when pressure is put on them. Then they are sore again when lifted. Heat is unbearable. The slightest movement is also unbearable.

Dosage: One Bryonia 30c, twice a day for three days.

Ledum Palustre

The soles are so sore that the person avoids stepping on them. Tenderness and some loose swelling in the pad behind the big toe. The pain is worse and the back of the foot itches at night, and the feet are very stiff on first rising in the morning. A strange symptom for Ledum is that the soles are most painful on walking upstairs. This person likes cold bathing and cold weather.

Dosage: One Ledum 6c, twice a day for three or four days.

Rhus Toxicodendron

Often the best remedy for sore and painful feet, especially when brought on by unusual and excessive exertion. The feet feel hot and painful, stiff and paralysed. Pain in the sole of the foot that the patient may describe as 'stitching' or similar. The pain could also be burning or aching. It is worse in the morning on waking and on rising, and after sitting in a chair and rising. First movement is painfully stiff, but continued movement eases the pain. The person is very restless, constantly moving the feet to ease the pain and to find a comfortable position.

Remember the basic symptoms for Rhus Tox., and bear in mind that they need not only be manifested in the injured part:

Hot, painful swelling, worse in the evening.

The pains are *tearing, shooting and stitching,* and the person *cannot rest.*

Worse at night.

Worse on first movement; better for continued movement.

Worse from exposure to wet and cold.

Worse at rest, which makes him restless.

Ailments brought on by overexertion.

Better from heat, hot bathing.

Dosage: You may find that you will use a range of potencies from 6c to 200c, and that some cases may need repeated doses.

Warning: Be careful not to repeat Rhus Tox., or indeed any remedy, too often or for too long without careful reconsideration of the case. Repeating the remedy daily for more than a week is not advisable. Always advise the person to stop taking the remedy once an improvement begins. Homoeopathic remedies continue to work for a long time even after the patient has stopped taking them. The lower potencies, i.e. 6c and 30c, can be repeated safely more often than the higher potencies such as 200c and upwards.

THE ANKLE

Between 13% and 15% of all sports injuries involve the ankle, and most of those involve the anterior talofibular ligament (Lachman and Jenner).

Ankle Sprains

Every ankle injury will require Arnica 6c as the first remedy. Repeat this every two hours for the first two days after injury.

The body's natural reaction to a sprain or strain is to produce splinting, or spasm in the local tendons, and swelling in the area. These immobilise the injured joint, and protect it from further damage. Swelling is the result of extravasation and inflammation, and inflammation is essential for healing. Too much inflammation produces too much swelling, which is counterproductive because it delays recovery. Arnica tends to restrict the body's reaction to almost exactly what is needed for speedy recovery.

It can work successfully even when given some time following an injury, as the following case shows.

CASE 15

Robert is a top-grade competitive skier. He injured his ankle in a fall during pre-season training in October, and had been diagnosed as having strained the talofibular ligaments of his right foot. He had received physiotherapy but the injury responded very slowly, and in February he still suffered too much pain to compete effectively. He was depressed by his lack of progress, and dissatisfied that he was not improving.

In my office he said that he was fine and probably did not need treatment. He also said he would like to compete in the British Championships that next March. I noticed that he kept his right foot and ankle well hidden whenever anyone moved around, and he agreed that he was very careful in case anyone touched his ankle. His ankle still felt bruised and sore. The last time he competed a friend noticed that he moaned as he negotiated each gate on the slalom course. His manager reported that he sat and thought, or brooded, for much of his time, and it was difficult to motivate him.

He preferred to be warm than cold, and he felt better when lying down.

Because of the time elapsed – five months between the injury and the consultation – I began treatment with Arnica 1M (the 1,000 potency), one tablet twice a day for three days.

The following week he started structured rehabilitation. He reported feeling much colder. His ankle felt worse when walking and when lying in bed. He was sleeping badly because he was restless, and wondered if he had overdone his training. He also reported some nausea and increased thirst for cold drinks.

I prescribed one Ruta 200c, twice daily for seven days. Rehabilitation was now going well and his ankle pain ceased, so after the first dose I advised him to stop taking the remedy. He competed in the British Championships and was free of pain.

Comment

You should expect to prescribe Arnica and Ruta for almost every ankle sprain because the injury almost always involves damage to ligaments. Arnica, given as soon as possible after the injury, will reduce the extravasation into the surrounding tissue and its resultant bruising, swelling and inflammation. Ruta has a specific affinity for tendons and ligaments, and will almost always assist the healing.

Immediate Treatment

Arnica

Give Arnica 30c as a first contact remedy in association with RICE. The patient should stop all exercise at first but gentle movement of the ankle can be resumed a few hours after injury. This will help to reduce swelling. Regular and frequent repetitions of static quadriceps exercises can be started almost immediately after injury. If ice cannot be tolerated then contrast bathing may be a more acceptable effective treatment.

The patient should be persuaded to rest, with the ankle higher than the hips, but with the whole leg supported with pillows while sitting and lying in bed. If the pain and swelling continue for more than a day, referral to a specialist for diagnosis may be recommended.

The routine prescription of Arnica immediately following injury, and of Ruta as a follow-up will have beneficial effects in most cases of ankle sprain.

Other remedies which may be useful for ankle sprains are:

Bellis Perennis

Bellis may be useful if Arnica does not seem to have worked, there is deep intense bruised pain, and the ankle feels as if it has an elastic bandage around it. The person feels chilled after being warm during exercise, but cold application to the ankle makes it better.

Dosage: One Bellis 30c, once or twice a day for two days.

Bryonia Alba

The person may feel that any movement at all is too painful to contemplate, even opening his eyes. Even the smallest movement of the injured part is painful. The joint is hot, red and swollen and pressure relieves the pain.
Dosage: One Bryonia 30c.

Phytolacca

The pain is like aching neuralgia in the ankle and in the tibia and toes. Cannot put the foot to the ground, and extending the ankle or leg is painful. Worse for motion. It may work in cases where Bryonia does not.
Dosage: One Phytolacca 30c.

Rhus Toxicodendron

The pain is tearing, shooting or stitching, worse at night and at rest. First movement painful but continued movement relieves the pain. Cannot rest, he gets up and walks around at night. Ankle swells after sitting or lying, and in the evening. Better after a hot bath.
Dosage: One Rhus Tox. 30c.

Ruta Graveolens

Ruta has a special affinity with ligaments and tendons, and should be used when you suspect strain, damage or inflammation in the ligaments or tendons of the ankle.

It will often be effective when the pain is the result of overuse, and when there is pain from the slightest physical exertion. Bruised, sore and aching pain felt in the bones of the ankle.

Similarly to Rhus Tox., there is pain on first movement that is eased by continued movement. So, how do you decide which to use?

The pains of Ruta are *bruised, sore and aching,* and the person is able to rest if kept warm, and after massage. The person needing Rhus Tox. cannot rest. Also compare the mental symptoms of each remedy in the Materia Medica in Chapter 10.

The person feels worse from cold, damp or wet weather, lying on the injured limb, sitting, exertion, ascending or descending steps. Better for warmth, rubbing, gentle motion, rest if he can find a comfortable position, lying on his back, but too much rest makes him worse.
Dosage: One Ruta 30c, three times daily for three days.

Strontium Carbonicum
The pain feels like gnawing into the bones, there is spasm and swelling of the ankle joint with oedema and it feels immobile and paralysed. The ankle is sprained and puffy, and continues to swell up long after injury.
Dosage: One Strontium Carb. 30c, three times a day for three days.

Second Stage of Recovery

The most important influence on recovery is exercise in the form of specific rehabilitation, preferably prescribed and supervised by a chartered physiotherapist. Non-weight-bearing and non-impact exercise should be substituted for running, walking, and other high impact sports, dance and aerobics. Use swimming, cycling, Pilates technique and sport, activity and dance-specific weight training to maintain cardiovascular fitness, and recommend flexibility, stretching and mobilising exercises. Balance exercises are important. Tai Chi and Chi Gong exercises may be recommended.

If there is residual pain and stiffness, and swelling occurs at the end of the day there are some remedies which can help.

Causticum
The ankle feels weak, walking is unsteady and there is tearing rheumatic pain in the joint. The pain may also be described as burning. There is a feeling that the tendons and ligaments are contracted, preventing movement. Some cracking may be felt in the joint, there may be cramps in the foot and calf. Legs are restless at night, pain like electric shocks in leg. Stiffness is worse from sitting and relieved by walking.
Dosage: One Causticum 30c, twice a day until the stiffness eases, but no longer than three days.

Chelidonium
The ankle, usually the right one, is very stiff and burning, and very sore to the touch. The stiffness is worse from moving but better after warm bathing. The pain is worse at 4 p.m. and 4 a.m. He is lethargic and drowsy but has trouble sleeping because he wakes at 4 a.m. Anxious, despondent and guilty about being injured.
Dosage: One Chelidonium 30c or 200c, twice daily for not more than seven days, or until the stiffness and pain ease.

Ruta Graveolens
This remedy may be needed for any ankle injury. Refer to the description above in 'First Stages of Recovery' (page 96). A higher potency may be more effective.
Dosage: One Ruta 30c or 200c, three times daily for three days.

Silica
This remedy has always been known for its ability to disperse scar tissue and adhesions. There are sticking pains and increased sensitivity to pain. Stiffness from scarring to tissue. Chronically weak ankles and feet. Leg feels paralysed, cannot walk. Lacks determination to recover and confidence, but may be obstinate about some things. Worse from cold and draughts, touch and pressure, better wrapping up warmly. May have sweaty and smelly feet.
Dosage: One Silica 30c tablet daily for two days. (But first note the warning on page 264.)

Sulphur
Ankle swollen, stiff and feels heavy. Feet are burning hot and red so that he wants them uncovered. The pains are burning and stitching. Walks unsteadily, and is much worse when standing. Worse from bathing of any sort, may be averse to washing. Untidy, talks about theories, which may be outrageous and far-fetched. Tends to be a hot person, better in the open air.
Dosage: One Sulphur 30c, three times a day for three days.

Rhus Tox. may also be needed. See Chapter 10 and page 93 above for details.

Long-Term Effects of Ankle Sprains

It is sometimes the case that a slight sprain of the ankle is much more painful than a serious ligament tear or even an avulsion fracture of either malleolus. The serious ligament tear may be dismissed from the accident clinic because there is no evident fracture. A serious sprain can, however, take months or even years to heal, as the following case illustrates. Joint instability is common following injury. It also demonstrates that the remedy chosen to fit the whole person will often be more effective than one for a specific injury, and that the correct remedy will work even years after the precipitating trauma.

CASE 16

Elizabeth sprained her right ankle when she was five years old, and consulted me when she was sixteen. She had become interested in hiking and mountain climbing, but the extra exertion was causing her problems. She had a continuous stabbing pain in the ankle, worse after a long walk in the hills. It was worse when she woke in the morning, and sometimes it woke her at night. The front part of her foot some-times swelled up. She was afraid she would never recover, and was 'fed up'.

Her ankle was worse from the touch of the bed clothes, and slightest pressure. She was very chatty, and talked a lot. Her mother described her as 'starting to talk when she wakes, and not stopping until she is asleep again.' Vivid dreams woke her most nights. She was a vegetarian, and disliked meat. She was afraid of wasps, describing them as 'evil', and feared all insects.

After Arsenicum Album 1M, one twice a day for three days, she reported back to me that her ankle had been 'better on more days than it is worse.' Six weeks later her ankle was better, and she was looking forward to increasing her walking and climbing.

The remedy that is chosen because it has an affinity for tendon and ligaments, or is a specific or local remedy, is not always the one that will cure most effectively. I chose Arsenicum Album on her mental, general and dream symptoms, and the chosen remedy also covered her ankle pain. This case is a good example of homoeopathy working on the whole person, not just on the presenting pathology.

The most effective homoeopathic sports injuries treatments will be those that follow the principles of homoeopathic prescribing.

Weak Ankles

As well as the remedies recommended for the second stage of recovery there are a few remedies which are specific for weakness in the ankles. These can be used in combination with strengthening, mobilising and balancing exercises prescribed by a chartered physiotherapist.

Calcarea Carbonica

Weak ankles which turn over too easily in heavily-built, overweight, flabby, fair children, young people and adults. Feet are always cold. Worse from exertion. Forgetful. Sour sweats about the head.
Dosage: One Calc. Carb. 30c tablet daily for two days.

Carbo Animalis

Weak ankles which turn over too easily, especially in children and young people. Foot and ankle are bluish-coloured. Feeble, has frequent colds and easy sprains. Ankle feels loose and dislocated.
Dosage: One Carbo Animalis 200c, twice a day for three days.

Natrum Carbonicum

Ankles weak, seem to dislocate and sprain easily, walks unsteadily. Trips over little obstructions or on rough ground. Burning pain in ankle, sole of foot tender, burns when walking. Cramp in ankle and foot. May be very thin or emaciated, cross, gloomy and irritable or indifferent. Dislikes thunderstorms. Much worse from heat.
Dosage: One Natrum Carb. 200c, twice a day for three days.

Nitric Acid

Weak ankles which crack when walking. Weakness may prevent walking. Tibia painfully sore, feeling of a splinter in the ankle. Ingrowing toenails, blue or yellow nails. Offensive foot sweat. Worse from touch, jarring, and cold. Better from steady pressure. Unwilling to work or make any effort, angry, curses and uses bad language.
Dosage: One Nitric Acid 200c, twice a day for three days.
Refer also to Rhus Tox., Silica and Sulphur above.

Prevention

Research has shown that an orthotic device reduces the risk of further ankle sprains in athletes and dancers who have suffered previous ankle injury. A suitably experienced physiotherapist or podiatrist can prescribe an orthotic (Davies and Taylor).

Fractures

What the layman commonly refers to as a 'broken ankle' is usually a fracture in the lower third of the tibia or fibula and really belongs to the lower leg. The repercussions such as swelling, pain and loss of mobility are manifested in the ankle joint. Homoeopathic treatment can be considered in two phases for fractures of the ankle such as avulsion fractures of the fibular or tibial malleolus or of both, and for dislocation of the ankle.

Phase 1:

Arnica

This of course is the first remedy and is necessary to counteract the trauma, to control the internal bleeding and to reduce the possibility of swelling and inflammation. The sooner it is taken, the shorter the recovery time will be.

Dosage: One Arnica 30c, three times daily for two days, will help. One can be taken anytime afterwards for relief of pain.

Aconite

Will help to relieve the immediate pain following trauma, especially when the person has been chilled, and if the injury occurred in cold weather. The pain is sticking, tearing, burning or tingling and the ankle feels deformed. The pain is worse at night, the patient is frightened by the injury or its circumstances, and anxious dreams and restlessness prevent sleep. Pale frightened face.

Dosage: One Aconite 30c, as frequently as necessary to control the pain. Stop when the pain ceases, or after three days.

Phase 2:

Symphytum

Once the fracture has been realigned or reduced and the bones reset, this remedy will encourage callus formation.

Dosage: One Symphytum 30c a day for two weeks.

Bryonia

This will help when the slightest movement, even of a distant part, causes pain in the injured joint. The swelling may be red, hot and painful to touch but – strangely – better when it is pressed, tightly bandaged or held. Look out for the characteristic mental symptoms of extreme irritability, wanting to be left alone, and wanting to go home before treatment is over or even before it begins. Bryonia will help when the person is reluctant to exercise while the lower leg is still immobilised, for example in a cast.

Dosage: One Bryonia 30c or 200c.

Kali Carbonicum

Aching, sciatic, shooting pains in the tibia and ankle which make the person bad-tempered and quarrelsome. (He is likely to be a bad-tempered person, but is normally able to keep this under control.)

Dosage: One Kali Carb. 30c.

Phytolacca

The pain is like aching neuralgia in the ankle and in the tibia and toes. Cannot put the foot to the ground, and extending the ankle or leg is painful. Worse for motion.

Dosage: One Phytolacca 30c, three times a day for two days.

Rhus Toxicodendron

Will alleviate pain when the ankle is rested, and when the pain is worse on first moving and relieved by continued movement. The ankle swells after the person has been resting or sitting for some time, and is more painful in cold, wet weather and at night. Look out for the typical mental symptoms of anxiety, depression and confusion, and the relief of pain from hot bathing. Rhus Tox. may be needed for some time following apparent recovery if the symptoms reappear.

Dosage: One Rhus Tox. 30c or 200c.

During recovery and rehabilitation the athlete or dancer may require remedies such as Rhus Tox., Bryonia and other remedies as indicated, especially when there is pain or stiffness as a result of rehabilitative treatment.

Achilles Tendon Rupture

When there is a partial or full rupture of the Achilles tendon there is a sudden severe pain which is similar to a blow to the calf. Typically, a doubles racquet player moves forward suddenly from the back of the court and thinks that his partner has hit his leg with his racquet.

Swelling and bruising may be present and the two ends of the tendon may leave a visible gap, but this is not always evident. The athlete or dancer falls at the moment of injury, and cannot walk. The most frequent cause of the injury is sudden strenuous activity such as sprinting, jumping or lunging when the muscle is either cold or very fatigued.

A ruptured tendon may need immobilisation for six weeks. In many cases it may be advisable to repair the rupture surgically. Treatment should be followed by rehabilitation which may be slow.

A partial rupture of the Achilles tendon produces sudden pain at the site of the injury. There is pain during physical activity and stiffness on moving before and after exercise. Local swelling is tender to touch, and the athlete experiences difficulty when the forward foot moves to the rear when walking.

Arnica
The injury is accompanied by bleeding into the tissues and can give rise to shock. It is necessary to limit the haemorrhage, exudates and subsequent inflammation, swelling and atrophy.
Dosage: Arnica in any potency available should be taken immediately and continued for three or four doses.

Ruta Graveolens
A partial rupture will take as long to recover as a full tear. Arnica is essential as a first remedy, followed by Ruta.
Dosage: Ruta 30c, one tablet twice daily for three days, will both relieve the pain and promote recovery.

Symphytum
If the tendon is repaired surgically, Symphytum 6c three times daily for two weeks will aid recovery. The same remedy will help recovery if the leg is immobilised.
Dosage: One Symphytum 6c, three times daily for two weeks.

Achilles Tendinitis and Peritendinitis

Pain and tenderness in the Achilles tendon is often caused by overuse and overload. Tendinitis may be caused by a small tear in the tendon, long distance running on hard surfaces, or by the back of a shoe or boot impinging on the tendon. Running in sand dunes and steeply uphill can be a cause. Dance class on unsuitable and hard surfaces may also cause Achilles tendinitis and peritendinitis. The conditions are common in dancers when there is overexertion of calf muscles with insufficient warm up and stretching. There is a danger of the condition recurring and, in older people, of the tendon developing cystic degeneration.

Peritendinitis is sometimes caused by changing to low-heeled shoes, or shoes or boots with rigid soles. The Achilles tendon does not have a sheath, and after overuse the surrounding connective tissue becomes inflamed and there may be crepitus.

There are two specific remedies for inflammation of the Achilles tendon and its surrounding tissue:

Sepia
The tendon feels too short and the legs are restless and twitching. The feet feel cold. The person feels better after violent strenuous exercise,

and from warmth. Hates cold. The typical mental and emotional symptoms of Sepia make it a remedy that may frequently apply to dancers (see Chapter 10).

Dosage: One Sepia 30c daily to reduce the inflammation.

Zinc

The pain is worse from heat, but better if the joint can be kept moving. Cannot keep the feet and legs still. The foot and toes feel swollen, even from a condition in the Achilles tendon, and there may be a sensation of itching or crawling over the skin which is better from rubbing or scratching.

Dosage: One Zinc 30c. (Rhus Tox. and Ruta may also be needed, according to the symptoms.)

Osteoarthritis

Although it is not due exclusively to injury, osteoarthritis may be a sequel of fractures and other ankle injuries. It occurs mainly in footballers, runners, dancers, and rugby players. Unfortunately the condition rarely becomes evident until the person reaches middle age. Its eventual onset may be precipitated by a return to full activity before the joint has reached total rehabilitation.

My files include many cases where the pain and disability of osteoarthritis have been relieved by homoeopathic medicines. There is no doubt that the earlier homoeopathic treatment is started, the better chance there is of success.

There are several homoeopathic remedies which have been used to treat people with osteoarthritis successfully. They cannot reverse the deterioration and pathological tissue change, but they can relieve the pain significantly.

Causticum

For arthritis following ankle injuries. Tearing, burning, rheumatic pain in the ankle, better from warmth of bed. Deformity. Tendons contracted. Cracking in joint. Electric shocks in leg. Restless legs at night. Worse dry cold air, windy weather, evening, and 3–4 a.m.

Dosage: One Causticum 30c, daily for three days.

Chamomilla

Violent rheumatic pains drive the person out of bed at night. Ankles give way. Feels as if walking on the ends of the bones. Cannot step on feet at night. Quarrelsome, cross and uncivil. Worse at night, and after drinking coffee.

Dosage: One Chamomilla 30c daily for three days.

Rhus Toxicodendron

Hot painful swelling of ankle. Feet swell in evening. Condyles of bones sore. Worse after sitting or lying. Worse during rest. Cannot find a comfortable position to rest or sleep. Must keep moving leg and ankle. Much worse if ankle is lain on. First movement is extremely painful, but continued movement relieves the pain. Worse on wet nights. Better from hot bathing. Depressed about the pain.

Dosage: One Rhus Tox. 30c daily for three days. It may be necessary to repeat the chosen remedy at intervals if the symptoms return.

Warning: In every case of ankle pain or sprain the athlete or dancer must discuss with an expert whether to continue. If there is the least doubt about his or her ability to continue then the decision must be to stop. Never play, perform or exercise 'through' the pain.

Rehabilitation should begin as soon as possible after the injury, using exercises to prevent muscle atrophy.

After injury, the return to full competition or performance should be delayed until the joint is mechanically fully recovered and entirely pain-free.

Using the appropriate homoeopathic remedies at every stage can help to avoid or delay the onset of osteoarthritis.

THE LEG

Shin Splints

'Shin splints' is a blanket description of persistent general pain over the front of the lower leg. The pain is most often felt on the lower inner side and is worse on dorsiflexion. It can be described as medial and anterior tibial soreness, may also be called tendinitis, and is usually caused by running. The pain is aggravated by exertion and gets worse during the exercise. There is almost always a history of increased activity such as increasing running mileage or dance performance, especially on hard or unsprung surfaces after a layoff, or by unaccustomed dancing, running or long walking. If the soreness is felt close to the shin bone or on the central ridge it may take longer to clear up, as the periosteum may be inflamed or damaged.

Stress fractures can mimic shin splints as both cause anterior shin pain. If pain persists for longer than an hour after cessation of exercise a stress fracture may be suspected and the patient referred for diagnosis and assessment accordingly. The pain from a stress fracture gets worse to the point where walking is painful and the pain persists even in bed.

Simple Test for a Stress Fracture

There is a simple test to confirm a stress fracture. A vibrating tuning fork placed on the centre of the painful area will cause tenderness in just one spot and signify a stress factor, whereas diffuse pain over a large area does not normally do so.

A great deal of research has been conducted into this condition, but its cause remains doubtful. In orthodox terms an inability to distinguish the cause of a condition prohibits the development of a satisfactory cure. Fortunately homoeopathy knows no such constraints, and the condition may be prescribed for simply by taking the symptoms and using them to choose the correct remedy.

The possibility that the pain was caused by trauma should be eliminated early in treatment. If trauma has been the cause, an immediate dose of Arnica in any potency should be given.

Treatment for Shin Pain

The athlete must rest to allow the acute condition to settle. An orthotic device which could successfully eliminate the condition may be prescribed by a podiatrist or orthotist.

The following homoeopathic remedies may help to reduce the pain and inflammation according to the symptoms manifested.

Agaricus Muscarius
Pain in the shin bone which appears gradually, and is worse when sitting. Feels as if needles are being pressed into the leg. Nervous twitching and then the leg becomes stiff and cold. Legs feel heavy, violent pains in the leg when crossing them. Itching and cramp in toes and feet. May talk a lot, change subjects rapidly and seem unable to concentrate. Worse in the morning and from cold, better from gentle motion.
Dosage: One Agaricus 30c. If the pain starts again, repeat the remedy.

Arnica
Dosage: One 30c tablet as soon as the pain is first felt.

Bryonia

If the person is averse to the least motion, not just of the injured leg, and the leg feels worse when elevated and with heat. The person is very irritable and wants to go home, despairs of getting better. There may be some redness and swelling around the painful area. Pain is better from pressure, such as tight bandaging, and he sits holding his leg.

Dosage: One Bryonia 30c.

Causticum

The pain is tearing and rheumatic, with burning. It may feel like an electric shock in the leg. The tendons feel contracted. The leg pain is much worse in the morning in bed, but, strangely, he feels better when he is warm in bed at night. The pain is much worse from getting cold, or having ice treatment. The person is very sensitive to the feelings of others, and very sympathetic. He will probably ask others about their problems rather than have his own dealt with, and will be overworked by dealing with others to the point of exhaustion.

Dosage: One Causticum 30c.

Phosphorus

Inflammation of the periosteum with tearing pain in the tibia. After exhaustion. Worse from any and every exertion. He is tottery and stumbles easily. His legs are heavy and his feet feel stuck to the floor. A very affectionate and sensitive person who cares much for others (but not as much as Causticum). Hates to be alone.

Dosage: One Phosphorus 30c.

Rhus Toxicodendron

Soreness in tibia at night and in bed. The pain is tearing, stitching and shooting, so bad at night that he cannot rest. The leg feels sore and bruised, and as if the flesh was torn from the bone. There may be inflammation and swelling. The person has to keep moving the leg because it feels better when he does, and so he is restless. First movement is painful, but continued movement eases the pain. The pain is worse on cold wet nights. Typical onset is after training, a run or dance session, cooling down and resting. Anxious and very depressed.

Dosage: One Rhus Tox. 30c.

Ruta Graveolens

This is the prime remedy for shin splints when the pain typically comes on after exercise, walking or running. The pain feels as if it is deep in the tibia and the person feels as if he should walk gently about indoors. Walking in the open air makes him worse. The pain may be eased during the day. The legs may feel weak, so weak that he cannot get out of a chair, and the ankle may be swollen. The leg feels bruised, sore and aching, and there is restlessness with intensely weary painfulness. The pains may be worse from lying, sitting and cold, and better from warmth. There may be hard nodules in the periosteum.

Look out for some depression about his condition, and a feeling that he will not improve. He may also be dissatisfied with himself and with his treatment. The Ruta patient may wake frequently from sleep after vivid confused dreams and yawn a lot, and stretch out his arms and hands.

Dosage: One Ruta 30c.

Stress Fracture of the Tibia

Stress fractures are among the most common of all sports injuries. They are most commonly found in the lower legs of runners who experience pain along the medial border of the tibia while training. The pain begins insidiously but as training continues it intensifies so much that running has to be reduced or stopped entirely. It is difficult to differentiate clinically between the inflammation of shin splints and the more severe stress syndrome or fracture. Pain from shin splints is usually present at the start of training but may disappear during exertion, only to return several hours later (see Rhus Tox.).

Gymnasts develop stress fractures of the wrist, and cricketers may develop them in the lumbar spine. Dancers develop them in the foot. They are partial or complete fractures of bone, and are called stress fractures because they are caused by repetitive strain during sub-maximal activity. The bone is unable to react favourably to the stress imposed by such activity.

The two types of stress fracture are fatigue fracture and insufficiency fracture. The former is most often encountered in runners. The latter is most often seen in post-menopausal women, and women with menstrual irregularity or disorder. Both types may be treated with homoeopathic remedies according to the presenting signs and symptoms.

Remedies for Stress Fracture of the Tibia

All the remedies listed above for shin splints can be considered for treating stress fractures according to the symptoms. If the pain persists for more than two weeks, the patient should be referred to a doctor for diagnosis.

Arnica

As soon as the pain becomes noticeable start taking Arnica. Arnica will be needed when the person tends to decline treatment or put it off and says, 'I'm OK. I'm fine. I don't need to be seen.' The pain starts after overexertion, or unusually increased activity or exercise – for example, when a recreational runner decides to increase his mileage from ten to twenty miles a week, and runs mainly on roads. The pain tends to start as a mild ache after a run, and he tries to 'run through it'. If there has been any trauma to the shin, Arnica is essential.
Dosage: One Arnica 30c.

Nitric Acid

The tibia is painfully sore, especially in a small spot. Look out for the person who indicates the pain by putting one finger on the spot. He does not want you to touch the spot because it hurts, but steady pressure ameliorates. Jarring hurts too. The ankles may be weak and crack when he walks. There may be a sensation of a splinter. Look out for discoloured, distorted toe nails. This may be the sort of person who feels driven to train, dance or work, often too hard, and becomes anxious and irritable if he cannot.
Dosage: One Nitric Acid 30c, three times a day for a week.

Rhododendron

Drawing, tearing pain in tibia. Feels as if he has a weight on his foot. Feet are cold. Better from heat, and better immediately he starts moving. (Rhus Tox. is better after the first few movements.) Slight exertion makes him exhausted and weak. Sensitive to storms and changing weather.
Dosage: One Rhododendron 30c, three times a day for a week.

Rhus Toxicodendron

Aching pain on first movement, relieved by continued movement. Pain during rest after exertion.
Dosage: One Rhus Tox. 30c taken before and after training.

Symphytum
When a stress fracture has been diagnosed, and while the person is resting.
Dosage: One Symphytum 30c taken three times a day for two weeks will promote healing.

Chronic Compartment Syndrome

Compartment syndrome occurs when muscle pressure increases to a level that inhibits blood flow within the muscle compartment. It is invariably exercise-induced, and the patient complains of aching or cramping pain, tenderness, tightness and possibly weakness in the anterior muscle or deep in the posterior muscles. The pain seems to come on after about twenty minutes of running or exercise, and is relieved when the exercise stops. There may be numbness and/or tingling along a nerve traversing the compartment.

The athlete should be discouraged from training 'through' the pain, as prolonged muscle soreness and pain can occur. There are two homoeopathic remedies that may help:

Hepar Sulphuris
Cramping, sore pain in muscle, very tender and sensitive to touch. Aggravated by running, especially in cold conditions and when the legs are cold. Relieved by rest. A very irritable, chilly person who notices draughts.
Dosage: One Hepar Sulph. 30c, taken before training.

Nitric Acid
Painful soreness in the region of the tibia. A sensation as if there is a splinter in the muscle, sore to touch. The muscle feels as if is sticking to nearby tissue. The jarring of running aggravates the pain. Anxious about the injury.
Dosage: One Nitric Acid 30c, taken before training.

Calf Muscle Tear

A tear in the gastrocnemius muscle is typically experienced by the older squash or tennis player or dancer who suddenly lunges, stretching his back leg in the process. He may describe the onset as being a sensation of 'unzipping' across the muscle. The injury is sometimes described as 'tennis leg', and even a mild tear will cause tenderness and seriously affect walking. A gross tear will generate considerable haemorrhage and subsequent swelling, pain and hardness. The foot cannot be dorsi-flexed and the typical walking action is that the non-weight-bearing foot cannot be brought forward of the other foot. There is a risk of further bleeding after about ten days when the newly formed scar tissue is very vulnerable to further tearing. The injury may be mistaken for a deep vein thrombosis, which could be life-threatening and must be referred to a doctor.

If older performers warm up with stretching exercises this disabling injury can largely be avoided.

CASE 17

A tennis player aged 45 was stretching well forward for a forehand stroke. He felt 'something give' in his rear leg. I saw him leave the court. He was limping badly, and unable to bring his left foot forward of his right when it was weight bearing. He had refused help, saying he was OK, and had tried to continue the game. He described the trauma as if a zip had been opened across his calf. 1 applied crushed ice with a crepe bandage in the changing room and gave him one Arnica 30c. There was still severe pain as he limped back to his car.

I advised RICE and hourly doses of Arnica. He rested and continued treatment for the following day. The day after he was able to walk again without much pain.

Arnica
Dosage: One Arnica 30c, three times a day until improvement begins. Two or three doses should also be taken about eight to ten days after injury to avoid the possibility of further bleeding.

Bellis Perennis
If Arnica does not relieve the pain, and the pain is deep in the muscle and unbearable. The Bellis person tells you he is injured and needs help, does not like the idea of ice if he is still hot from activity, but finds that the ice treatment is very effective and relieves the pain.
Dosage: One Bellis 30c every few hours for a day. Depending on the symptoms, Ruta and/or Rhus Tox. may also be required until fully recovered. Bryonia will help the patient to move the limb if he finds this difficult or painful. Refer to Chapter 10 for details.

THE KNEE

CASE 18

James is a recreational skier. Towards the end of his holiday he fell on a very steep slope. He thinks he may have hit a rock with his knee. It was very painful. He limped back to the valley and packed ice around the joint. His knee was too swollen to ski the following day, and he ended his holiday very disconsolate and depressed. The day after his return he saw his GP who diagnosed a torn medial ligament, and prescribed an immobilising strapping, mild pain killers and crutches.

James' wife is a patient in my practice. She is a very determined woman. Despite his reluctance to make a fuss and assurances that he was OK, she persuaded him to call me. I gave him Arnica 30c to take every hour for a day, and followed this with Ruta 30c, three times in one day. He immediately felt less depressed, and allowed his wife to remove his strapping and take back the crutches. With physiotherapy and exercises he was back at work and exercising fully within a week.

The knee is the most frequent source of injury from sports, especially in contact sports and running. The former produces traumatic injury, the latter, overuse injury. The knee is the second most frequent site of injury in dancers. Incorrect technique and outward rotation produces pain, swelling and inflammation of the ligaments. Pain from knee injury may be referred to the hip from the knee. An accurate history of the condition is essential.

Much has been written and discussed about knee injuries, enough to make the knee almost a speciality of its own. In homoeopathic terms the various pathological causes of pain, immobility, stiffness, swelling and other disease produce symptoms that will help you to choose a remedy to help the patient heal more effectively. Specific diagnosis may be less important than how the injury occurred, when the pain is worse, the type of pain and how the patient feels about his injury. We will, however, look at potentially helpful remedies through the main injuries that will bring athletes to your clinic.

Anterior Knee Pain

Anterior knee pain can be due to many conditions. The diagnosis may be chondromalacia patella, patellar malalignment syndrome, infrapatellar tendinitis, Osgood-Schlatter disease or similar. Whatever the pathological diagnosis may be, you can prescribe homoeopathic remedies according to the symptoms presented by the patient. Over the years homoeopaths have found certain remedies to be effective for specific conditions, but these will only work when the symptoms fit.

Patellofemoral Pain (Runner's Knee)

Runners notice an insidious onset of an ill-defined ache localised in the anterior knee behind the knee cap. The pain may sometimes be felt along the medial or lateral edge of the patella and is aggravated by downhill running. There may be complaints of swelling or of sudden weakness with a feeling that the knee 'gives way'.

This anterior knee condition affects the posterior surface of the patella and may be incorrectly seen as a precursor to osteoarthritis, or as a sign of cartilage damage. A more apt description would be to call it 'runner's knee'. It happens to runners who have increased their mileage, new joggers and runners, marathon runners, young athletes and dancers, tennis players, footballers, and dancers.

Typically the performer feels pain in or behind the patella and decides to 'work through it'. After a strenuous bout of activity, the pain characteristically develops after rest following activity the day before. The knee becomes stiff after being in one position for a long time while sitting or lying. It is very painful on standing up from sitting. Squatting and kneeling are painful, and the pain is worse when walking downhill or down stairs.

Runner's knee may arise from muscle imbalances, unusual foot biomechanics and imbalance, one leg being abnormally shorter than the other, or a wider than normal pelvis. Orthotics prescribed by a podiatrist or orthotist can help to resolve all these conditions.

Rest from painful activities is essential. The person may benefit from static exercises that brace the quadriceps, alternative, non-weight-bearing activities like swimming and cycling as long as they do not produce pain, and bandaging, rest and elevation.

The homoeopathic remedies listed overleaf will probably eliminate the need for anti-inflammatory drugs, but if the pain and swelling are still troublesome after some days, refer to a professional homoeopath, who may suggest other remedies.

Arnica

Give Arnica if there is bruising pain or aching, and to help overcome the trauma. Look out for the person who says, 'I'm OK. I'm fine,' is sensitive to touch, and wants to be left alone.

Dosage: One Arnica 30c, three times a day for two days.

Bryonia

There is hot red swelling around the patella and the person does not want to move his knee or any other part of his body, preferring to lie quietly. Better from pressure on the knee, likes to have it bound up tightly and kept cool. The knee feels weak and bends under him. It is effective in conjunction with Rhus Tox. (see below) if the pain is worse on first movement, then eased by continuous movement, and then gets worse again with continued movement.

Dosage: One Bryonia 30c, three times a day for not more than two days, or until the pain stops.

Calcarea Carbonica

This remedy can be useful when the cause of the condition is suspected to be pronation of the feet from weak ankles. The pain is worse when rising from a seat and when sitting. There may be weakness and trembling in the limb, and the feet may be cold and flabby. The person may be fair and well built, prone to putting on weight too easily, and hates cold. He is worse from exertion. If you bind up this person's knee he will become worse.

Dosage: One Calc. Carb. 30c, three times daily for a week can help to relieve the pain. Stop when the pain eases.

Chelidonium

Pain, burning, and stiffness in the right knee, especially in the patellar tendon. The knee is very sore to touch, and the limb feels heavy and paralysed. Worse at 4 a.m. and 4 p.m., and from motion. Tired. Better from hot bathing.

Dosage: One Chelidonium 30c.

Nitric Acid

Pain in the patella that makes walking difficult, and extends to the tibia. Worse from cold, touch and jarring. The pain is like a splinter. Look out for someone who may be taciturn and quarrelsome.

Dosage: One Nitric Acid 30c.

Rhus Toxicodendron

The knee feels worse on first movement, rising from a seat or in the morning, but is better with continuous movement. There is sore pain and stiffness at night so that the person cannot find a pain-free position in which to sleep. The knee is worse when laid on. The person is restless and exhausted by the restlessness. The pain may come on after strenuous activity, and especially at night during wet, cold weather. Better from hot bathing and from heat in general. Look out for the person who is anxious and depressed about the injury.

Dosage: One Rhus Tox. 30c.

Zinc

Pain in the patellar tendon while walking. Feet and legs are very restless. Cannot keep them still. The pain comes on after a very exhausting performance or event, and the person feels totally exhausted, both mentally and physically. Likes the knee to be bound up tightly. Hard pressure and massage relieve the pain. He moans or calls out with pain, and may repeat the questions you ask before replying.

Dosage: One Zinc 30c.

Haematoma

Arnica

Arnica 6c, 30c, or 200c, given immediately, or soon after the traumatic injury, and repeated for six doses will prevent bruising, haemorrhage into the bursa or capsule, inflammation and subsequent problems.

Infrapatellar Tendinitis

Overuse such as long-distance running, fell-running, hopping, kicking , dance or squatting may cause inflammation and pain in the infra-patellar tendon. This is particularly at risk after strenuous exertion, and during severe exertion, especially squatting with weights, when cold and not warmed up well. The pain does not usually prevent exertion, but continued use may lead to scar tissue which in turn produces adhesions, and possibly bone spurs. Early diagnosis and treatment are obviously desirable.

The patient should not participate in activities that cause pain, and should stretch the quadriceps gently but effectively as part of a good warm-up before exercise. Take whichever of the following homoeo-pathic remedies fits the symptom picture most closely.

115

Arnica
See page 114.

Rhus Toxicodendron
Very stiff on first movement (see above). Pain in the head of the tibia, worse at night in bed, and after walking.
Dosage: One Rhus Tox. 30c, three times a day for two or three days. See also Chelidonium and Zinc in the 'Runner's Knee' section (pages 114 and 115).

Ruta Graveolens
Stiffness, soreness, aching, bruised pain in the tendon with great restlessness, bursitis, cracking in the knee. Pains are worse when walking in the open air. The knees are weak and give way when descending and ascending stairs. Comes on as a result of overexertion, made worse by cold, lying, sitting and more exertion, and better from warmth and massage. The person seems tired, cranky, moody, fretful and depressed about his condition.
Dosage: One Ruta 30c, three times a day for two or three days to relieve the pain and to assist healing.

Osgood-Schlatter Disease

This painful condition affects active, sporting adolescents and dancers who may have grown recently. Its cause is repetitive strenuous exertion that causes pain, stiffness, inflammation and swelling in the knee, especially in the tubercle of the tibia, which may become detached. The pain is worse when the knee is stressed during repetitive activity, when kneeling, running, jumping and descending stairs.

Rest from all activity except for moderate walking and non-competitive swimming and cycling, together with ice treatment, will often reduce the symptoms in three weeks or so. If the pain is not relieved in three weeks, immobilisation may be needed.

Causticum
The pain is tearing and rheumatic with burning. Worse when sitting and better from continued walking. The tendons feel contracted with cracking and tension in the knee, especially when descending. Stiffness felt in the hollow of the knee. The pain is much worse in the morning in bed, but, strangely, he feels better when he is warm in bed at night. The pain is much worse from getting cold, or having ice treatment. The

person is very sensitive to the feelings of others, and very sympathetic. He will probably ask others about their problems rather than have his own dealt with.

Dosage: One Causticum 30c as needed to relieve the pain. If it is effective, it can be used throughout the time it takes to heal.

Natrum Muriaticum

Wrenching pain in knee, like an ulcer in the tubercle, when walking and standing. Restlessness and jerking of legs, cracking in knees during movement. Worse from heat and exertion. Hates sympathy.

Dosage: One Natrum Mur. 30c, as necessary for pain.

Rhus Toxicodendron

See above. Especially if there is cracking in the knee, if the pain follows unusual exertion, and on first movement.

Ruta Graveolens

See opposite.

Symphytum

If fragmentation of the tubercle is suspected or diagnosed. There is excessive neuralgic pain, stitching pain when bending the knee, worse from touch. This remedy acts as a bone healer. Its old country name is 'knitbone'.

Dosage: One Symphytum 30c, three times daily for two weeks.

Collateral Ligament Injuries

The medial collateral ligament (MCL) helps keep the knee stable by resisting external rotation of the tibia and valgus forces. MCL sprains are tension injuries that are usually the result of a blow to the lateral aspect of the knee. Orthodox treatment includes lightweight support and aggressive early rehabilitation. Sometimes, in combined injuries, the cruciate ligaments require surgical reconstruction. Braces may be worn, but their effectiveness is uncertain.

An application of external force to the leg and twisting in extension, during a tackle in rugby, or resistance to rotational force are often causes of MCL injury. When, for example, a footballer is tackled while his boot is fixed in the pitch, enough stress is produced on the ligament to cause traumatic stretching or tearing to the medial ligament. Injuries to the lateral ligament are not as frequent as to the medial. The same homoeopathic remedies will work for both.

CASE 19

A footballer aged 26 had received a full-weight tackle on his left leg while it was extended. He felt something tear in his knee, and had to leave the field. The knee was strapped up with an elastic bandage, but he felt nauseous, cold and shocked. He felt too bad to join in when his team mates had a post-match beer, and lay in the dressing room with his leg elevated.

The following day his knee was swollen, painful and immobile. He was unwilling to move, and simply wanted to lie still.

He consulted his GP, who diagnosed a ligament tear. He prescribed an anti-inflammatory drug and strapping to immobilise the joint. The club physiotherapist called me about him because a few days later he was still in shock and nauseous and wanted to go back to work. I met him at the club, and his first words were, 'I'm OK. I just want to get back to work, and start playing again.' He was very unwilling to have anyone treat his knee. He sat with his leg elevated on a chair. He totally rejected the physio's suggestion of static quadriceps exercises. He had not slept well since the injury because he felt bruised all over, and the bed was too hard. He moved his leg away as if to protect it whenever anyone came close.

I gave him one Arnica 200c immediately, and told him to take one later for the shock, nausea and pain. He allowed the physio to examine his knee and to treat it a few minutes later. He was able to start static exercises the following day, but was still reluctant to move much. One Bryonia 30c helped him to move without pain.

Three weeks later he was fully weight-bearing but his joint mobility was still less than 90 degrees of flexion without pain. There was a notch on the ligament, The swelling was almost totally reduced. His leg felt weak, and as if it would give way when he stood. He was 'fed up' with being injured, and was not sleeping well because of pain in his knee. He felt it would 'go out' if he moved in bed.

He took one Ruta 30c, three times daily for one week, and continued physiotherapy. The improvement was dramatic. Three days after starting Ruta his mobility improved to more than 90 degrees and he could begin active weight-bearing exercise. He was playing again two weeks later.

If this player had had ice applied and taken Arnica immediately after injury he could have avoided the shock and much of the swelling and immobility. Recovery would have been even quicker.

First-Stage Remedies (immediately post-trauma)

Arnica
Dosage: One Arnica 30c, as soon as possible after the injury. Give two or three doses an hour apart.

Bellis Perennis
If Arnica does not relieve the pain after two or three doses. The person cannot tolerate cold in any form. The knee feels better from heat and hot applications. The pain and bruising is deeper than in Arnica and may be felt up the front of the thigh. He moves impulsively.
Dosage: One Bellis 30c, two or three doses.

Bryonia
Even the *idea* of moving is painful. He does not want to move, talk, change position, go to the toilet, wash or anything. He would like a hot bath because it will improve his knee, but the idea of getting to the bathroom is too painful. Although his knee is painful, hard pressure on it and tight bandaging relieves the pain. You will find this remedy will be helpful for most traumatic injuries where the pain is immobilising.
Dosage: One Bryonia 30c will help him to get moving. Repeat as necessary.

Second-Stage Remedies (longer-term remedies)

Rhus Toxicodendron
Give Rhus Tox. at any time during the recovery if the symptoms fit and the person needs it, especially if you suspect that adhesions are slowing recovery.

If the knee feels worse on first movement, rising from a seat or in the morning, but is better with continuous movement, there is sore pain and stiffness at night so that the person cannot find a pain-free position to sleep, and the knee is worse when laid on. The person is restless and exhausted by the restlessness. The pain may come on at night during wet cold weather, and is better from hot bathing and from heat in general. Look out for the person who is anxious and depressed about his injury.
Dosage: One Rhus Tox. 30c, three times daily for two or three days.

Ruta Graveolens

The person seems tired, cranky, moody, fretful and depressed about his condition. I have found that Ruta has the immediate effect of making the person believe he will recover when he is most depressed and despondent about his injury. He begins to want to get better, to exercise and have treatment, and he adopts a much more positive attitude. Stiffness, soreness, aching, bruised pain in the ligament with great restlessness. Pains are worse when walking in the open air. Knees are weak and give way when descending and ascending stairs. The condition is aggravated by cold, lying, sitting and exertion, and better from warmth and massage.

Dosage: One Ruta 30c, three times a day for two or three days.

Long-Term Effects of Knee Injury

If the injury continues to bother the athlete or dancer and affect his performance long after he should have recovered, the following remedies may prove useful.

Calcarea Carbonica

The knee may continue to swell following exertion some time after the injury, perhaps when the athlete or dancer has started activity again. He or she may express doubts about recovery, and becomes depressed about it. May be naturally flabby and inclined to put on weight easily, but works hard at fitness. Look out for cold feet and a flabby handshake.

Dosage: One Calc. Carb. 30c. Two doses will help to reduce and prevent swelling. One Calc. Carb. 30c before each match, class, training session or performance until the possibility of further swelling has disappeared.

Calcarea Fluorica

This a very specific remedy for pain and tenderness over the medial ligament associated with calcification and possibly ossification in the ligament. It is sometimes needed following repeated medial ligament sprains or haematomae from direct blows. The pain is worse after rest and relieved by moving a little (not as much as Rhus Tox.), and by warm applications.

Dosage: One Calc. Fluor. 30c or 200c, daily for not more than two or three weeks.

Chelidonium
Continuing stiffness and swelling in the right knee, worse from exertion. This athlete or dancer may be lethargic in his or her approach to training and playing, and inclined to be 'liverish' in the morning.
Dosage: One Chelidonium 30c.

Pulsatilla
Continued swelling, comes and goes without pattern. Hot and painful swelling, or cold and white. Pain comes and goes, and may wander to other limbs or places. The athlete or dancer is disinclined to stand for long. Dislikes warm, stuffy rooms. Much better in the open air.
Dosage: One Pulsatilla 30c.

Silica
This remedy can help to eradicate scar tissue, and may be used to release adhesions. The athlete or dancer may have lost self-confidence after injury, and believes he cannot succeed or perform well. He may hide this feeling with obstinacy and a kind of determination. Very sensitive to drafts, and likes to wrap up well. Rough, yellow, brittle nails.
Dosage: One Silica 30c.

Warning: Do not give Silica above the 6c potency if the patient has synthetic tissue of any sort in his body. A replacement hip, or a polytetrafluoroethylene (PTFE) repair to a cruciate ligament, even a pacemaker, may be rejected following Silica in potency of 30c or higher.

Strontium Carbonicum
Continued oedema long after knee injury. Gnawing pain into the bones. Sprained and puffy knees and ankles. Burning, gnawing pains. Limb feels immobile and weak.
Dosage: One Strontium Carb. 30c to reduce the swelling.

Iliotibial Band Syndrome (Snapping Band)

Lateral knee pain is a frequent problem among distance runners. Iliotibial band syndrome is the most common cause and results from the iliotibial band rubbing as it slides over the lateral femoral epicondyle.

There is a developing feeling of tightness and often a burning pain over the lateral aspect of the knee while running. The pain typically comes on after the same distance has been run each time. Walking may not be painful, although climbing or descending stairs may be.

Running long distances on a cambered road where the feet are always angled to one side may cause friction between the iliotibial band and the axis of the knee. The iliotibial tract may become swollen and thickened. Pain may also occur over the trochanteric bursa. In severe cases there may be a sensation of a 'snapping band' on the lateral side of the knee. Look at the possible causes such as worn-down shoes, cambered road running, or varus which could be corrected with orthotics, and eliminate them if possible. Raked stages may contribute to the condition in dancers.

Arnica
If the cause is overexertion such as a recent major increase in running distance or speed work, or a major event such as a marathon.
Dosage: One Arnica 30c.

Rhus Toxicodendron
Use Rhus Tox. 30c if the pain is worse on first movement but relieved by continued movement, and the patient is restless, anxious and depressed.
Dosage: One Rhus Tox. 30c daily for three days.

Ruta Graveolens
If gentle motion ameliorates the pain and the legs give out when rising from a chair, and if the patient is depressed and dissatisfied.
Dosage: One Ruta 30c, three times a day for three days.

Sticta Pulmonaria
Sticta 30c may be useful if the pain is in the hip and due to bursitis. See the details in Chapter 10 and below under 'Bursae and Bursitis' (pages 126–8).
Dosage: One Sticta 30c daily for three days.

Torn Meniscus

The most common meniscus tear is in the medial meniscus, and is usually the result of twisting force on the weight-bearing leg that causes a femoral condyle to shear the fibrocartilage of the meniscus. It may be associated with a tear of the collateral ligament. In footballers and dancers there can also be cruciate ligament damage. These are shocking and devastating injuries to a professional that can destroy a career.

There is typically a locking of the knee due to the presence of loose material getting trapped between joint surfaces. The knee is commonly locked in a flexed position. The onset is sudden, and pain is deep within the knee. The patient may describe a feeling of 'giving way'. Effusion may be extensive and haemarthrosis may result if there is ligament damage. This can give rise to serious muscle atrophy.

Immediate basic first aid and referral for medical attention are essential.

Arnica
This remedy will limit the effusion and haemarthrosis, and the subsequent swelling. It will reduce the pain, prevent shock and limit the subsequent atrophy.
Dosage: One tablet of Arnica, any potency, immediately and three times daily for three days after injury.

For bruising, swelling and pain use Ruta, Bryonia, Ledum and Bellis according to the symptoms outlined above. The following remedies may also help:

Guaiacum
The knee remains flexed and there is tearing pain when attempting extension. The least movement of the leg will be very painful, and there is a reluctance to move. Heat and touch makes it worse. Worse when sitting, and in the morning. Look out for yawning and stretching, some obstinacy and fixed ideas.
Dosage: One Guaiacum 30c.

Lycopodium
Locked knee that has tearing pain preventing extension. The person describes the knee as giving way suddenly. It is relieved by heat, and he is not so reluctant to move. He feels better generally from heat but dislikes a warm room. Pressure hurts. Wakes feeling bad, and may be angry about the injury. This remedy is useful, especially for injuries to the right knee.
Dosage: One Lycopodium 30c.

Torn Cruciate Ligament

The anterior cruciate ligament may be injured in sport and dance. The performer has usually participated in running, jumping or skiing and has stopped suddenly and fallen with a twisting movement. He may have attempted a 'cutting' tackle in football. The combination of abduction and rotation is similar to that which causes meniscus and medial ligament damage, and the three injuries often form what is known as the 'unhappy triad'.

Swelling is often immediate as the result of haemarthrosis. Within twenty-four hours a minor tear of the cruciate ligament can produce a tense swelling. Arnica in any potency, given immediately and followed by several doses, will help to keep the effusion and swelling to the minimum and reduce shock.

Homoeopathic treatment for all three of the 'unhappy triad' should be according to the manifested symptoms. Please refer to the previous sections on collateral ligaments and meniscus for details of the most commonly recommended remedies. Give Ruta, Rhus Tox. and Bryonia as necessary, plus Symphytum to help the tendons, ligaments and cartilage to repair. There are two remedies that are almost specific to the unusual symptoms of this condition:

Calcarea Fluorica
This remedy can promote the recovery of damaged fibrous tissue.
Dosage: Take one Calc. Fluor. 6x three times daily for as long as necessary, but for not more than a month.

Phosphorus
If during recovery there is a feeling of looseness in the knee so that it feels as if it would dislocate, burning pain or soreness in a small spot, extreme stiffness and weakness, all of which are worse from exertion, this remedy will help. The knee will be much worse if he lies on it, and from cold, and the pain will come on after he has been at work. This person is very sensitive, anxious, and seeks sympathy.
Dosage: One Phosphorus 30c.

CASE 20
This patient is an older woman who is very fit. She runs, weight-trains, and practises Tai Chi. During one stretching session she decided to increase the flexibility of her knees and sat back on her heels forcefully for two sets of two minutes each. She experienced some stiffness in her right knee on standing.

The following day she had some pain in the medial posterior aspect of the right knee that was noticeable on rising from a seat. She felt her knee give way when she dismounted from her bicycle. In her next Tai Chi session certain twisting movements gave her pain and she felt again that the knee would give way. She described the pain as being like a splinter inside her knee.

It was a minor condition. She thought it did not merit a sports medicine consultation. She mentioned it to me during a homoeopathic consultation for another matter.

I suspected a strain of the posterior cruciate ligament due to the unusual forced flexion of the knee, and prescribed Ruta for the acute condition. She telephoned soon after to report that there was little change.

Comment
I looked at her case again. As she was a longstanding patient I already knew a lot about her; that she disliked milk and dairy products, and cold air, that she took up Tai Chi later in life because it gave her exercise without jarring and that she enjoyed the smooth, gliding nature of the exercise. She belonged to a type of person who seems driven to work and exercise as if afraid that once they stop they will give up altogether. I decided to prescribe Nitric Acid 200c three times daily for two days or until the pain eased. This was one of the remedies under consideration for her constitutionally.

After one day of Nitric Acid 200c she reported that the pain had gone, and she later went on to improve in other aspects of her health.

The only matching knee symptom for Nitric Acid in this patient's condition was a splinter-like pain in the hollow of the knee, but the remedy cured her acute condition. This case is a good example of a remedy prescribed according to mental and general symptoms. It is not normally associated with weakness and giving way on standing and after exercise, or with pain in the hollow of the knee. Successful homoeopathic prescribing takes patience, a knowledge of the remedies, an ability to observe and listen to the patient and an open mind.

Before Surgery to the Knee
The patient should take one Arnica 30c before the operation. If he is very apprehensive about the operation, has great anxiety about it and is even very frightened, one Aconite 200c or 1M will help to calm the nerves.

After Surgery to the Knee
Arnica
Dosage: One 30c tablet as soon as possible after surgery.

Bryonia
If the patient is reluctant to move, and to ease the first movements after surgery. This should be given routinely postoperatively for surgery to the knee.
Dosage: One Bryonia 30c.

Ruta Graveolens
To help healing of the ligament.
Dosage: One Ruta 30c, three times daily for two weeks.

Staphysagria
This remedy has a reputation for healing cuts from sharp instruments and for healing lacerated fibrous tissue. The knee feels beaten and painful.
Dosage: One Staphysagria 30c, three times following the operation.

If swelling returns some time after the operation, Rhus Tox., Calc. Carb., Chelidonium, Pulsatilla or other remedies as indicated by the symptoms may be necessary. For details see the section above on recurring swelling (page 120).

Bursae and Bursitis

Falls where the patella hits a hard surface can cause traumatic effusion or haemorrhage in the prepatellar bursa. A kick to the knee, or frequent kneeling such as performed by Aikido players and carpet layers can also cause the condition that is still sometimes called 'housemaid's knee'.

Haemorrhage can cause inflammation and swelling, and septic bursitis may result from secondary infection if the skin over the bursa is broken by laceration or a puncture wound. I experienced this before I knew about homoeopathy. Jumping down from a ledge during a climbing trip on limestone, my knee hit the rock and a sharp needle of limestone pierced the bursa. Within minutes the knee was swollen and very painful. I could walk only with difficulty, and felt shocked. In two or three hours I was becoming septicaemic. It resulted in a short stay in hospital and my climbing was curtailed for several weeks. I am sure, now, that if I had known about Arnica and used it immediately, followed by Sticta, I could have avoided these serious sequelae.

When choosing a homoeopathic remedy it is best to consider the location and the type of pain and modalities, such as 'worse kneeling', 'worse from first movement', etc., and to choose one of the remedies already discussed above. There are a few remedies which are specific for bursitis. Remember too that if there is a history of trauma the treatment should always start with Arnica.

Remedies for Bursitis

Baryta Carbonica
If someone complains of pain in the knee when kneeling, and you suspect that bursitis in its early stages, it is possible to prevent its development with a few doses of Baryta Carb.
Dosage: One Baryta Carb. 30c, three times daily for one week.

Natrum Muriaticum
This is almost specific for 'housemaid's knee'. Any pressure on the knee is painful. There is trembling, tingling and numbness. The condition comes on periodically, every day at a certain time, probably 9 to 11 a.m. every other day, or even every week. It is made worse by heat, and is better in the open air. This person is very reserved and detests fuss or consolation.
Dosage: One Nat. Mur. 30c, three times daily for one week.

Silica
Silica is specific for enlargement of the prepatellar bursa and any inflammatory knee conditions. It will work better if other Silica symptoms are also present. You should look out for very sweaty and smelly feet, a feeling of paralysis in the legs when walking, a tendency towards cramps in the calves in the evening after training, and slow healing of cuts. The person dislikes cold, fresh air, and draughts, and, of course, pressure on his knee makes it worse. He can seem to lack confidence in his own ability, but at other times can be quite determined and even obstinate.
Dosage: One Silica 30c, three times daily for one week.

Warning: Do not give Silica above the 6c potency if the patient has synthetic tissue of any sort in his body. A replacement hip, or a polytetrafluoroethylene (PTFE) repair to a cruciate ligament may be rejected following Silica in high potency.

Sticta Pulmonaria

Sticta is usually necessary when the swelling feels especially spongy after a fall or blow. The swollen joint has red spots. The pain is stabbing and cutting. Sticta is another specific remedy for 'housemaid's knee'. The knee is better from pressure, whereas Nat. Mur. and Silica are worse from pressure. Sticta is worse from touch and motion and gets worse as the day goes on. Sponginess is the best indication for this remedy.

Dosage: One Sticta 30c, repeated as necessary.

Posterior Knee Pain

Pain and swelling behind the knee may result from a tendon strain, tendinitis or a Baker's cyst. Pain may be caused by a strain to the hamstrings, popliteal or gastrocnemius muscles. If the cause is an obvious overuse or trauma, Arnica should be taken first. One of the following remedies will help healing.

Causticum

Stiffness in the hollow of the knee with cracking and a feeling of tension. The pain is tearing and rheumatic with burning. Worse when sitting and starting to walk. The tendons feel contracted with cracking and tension in the knee, especially when descending. The pain is much worse in the morning in bed. The pain is much worse from getting cold, or having ice treatment.

Dosage: One Causticum 30c three times daily for a maximum of one month.

Magnesia Carbonica

This is a specific remedy for Baker's cyst when there is swelling in the popliteal, and especially for the left knee. Cannot put the left foot to the ground. Feels better walking about in the open air despite the pain. The pain seems to be worse every other day, and is better from motion.

Dosage: Three Mag. Carb. 30c daily for two or three days.

Rhus Toxicodendron

This is the first choice remedy for the condition if there is pain and swelling behind the knee when bending, extending and walking, especially on first movement but relieved by continued motion. Pain in the back of the thigh causing limping. The cause is likely to be overuse, and increased exertion. The pain will be worse at night and during rest. Rest is almost impossible because he has to keep moving to relieve the pain.

Dosage: One Rhus Tox. 30c three times daily for one week.

THIGH, HIP AND GROIN INJURIES

Hamstrings

Acute hamstring tears occur most commonly in sprinting, whether in an athletics event or when a player sprints as part of another sport. They account for many lost performances and layoffs by sports people, and are most likely to have occured when warm-up and stretching have been inadequate and in cold weather.

The tear is usually in the belly of the muscle and is often accompanied by local haemorrhage. There is often tenderness and pain on movement. Movement, especially extension, may be inhibited by the pain and swelling.

One danger is that scar tissue may form which predisposes the muscle to further tears, and makes the condition chronic. Physiotherapy, gentle stretching, and a prohibition from competition until the injury is completely healed are essential. Early treatment will drastically reduce the length of the recovery period. RICE will help, but homoeopathic treatment immediately after the incident will prevent haemorrhage and its sequelae.

Arnica
The athlete must take Arnica in any potency at once and repeat it frequently for the first few hours. This will reduce the possibility of haemorrhage, swelling and immobility and the subsequent development of scar tissue. Recovery may not then take months. If Arnica does not seem to work after one or two doses, use Bellis instead. (See also 'Calf Muscle Tear', page 110.)
Dosage: One Arnica 6c, 30c or 200c, immediately and one every hour for up to one day.

Arsenicum Album
Stiffness and lameness with pain behind the thigh. He cannot extend the knee. It is a burning pain, but heat relieves it. He has to move his feet constantly, and may move from place to place. Is much worse from cold

in any form. Worse at 1 or 2 a.m. Very sensitive, fastidious, irritable and careful with money. Believes he cannot recover, and forecasts all kinds of disaster as a result of the injury.

Dosage: One Arsenicum 30c three times daily will help recovery. Stop the remedy when the pain, stiffness and lameness begin to ease.

Rhus Toxicodendron

If there is stiffness, better from heat and from continued movement, but worse on first movement. Typically the athlete has warmed up well, then cooled down, and then gone into a violent sprint or surge of effort.

Dosage: One Rhus Tox. 30c.

Ruta Graveolens

If there is soreness and stiffness in the muscle. Worse from cold, damp, lying and sitting. Better from warmth, rubbing, motion. The person is uncomfortable sitting with his leg on the edge of a seat. He is dissatisfied and depressed by his injury.

Dosage: One Ruta 30c three times a day for three days. Then stop. Repeat if necessary.

Symphytum

This remedy will promote healing of the tear.

Dosage: One Symphytum 30c daily for two weeks.

Quadriceps

Intramuscular haematoma, 'deadleg' or 'charley horse', results from a blow or kick to the thigh in contact sports. The muscles will have become engorged with blood before and during a match and a blow ruptures blood vessels, causing a massive extravasation of blood. This may be as much as a litre, distending the fascial compartment of the muscle. This impairs flexion of the knee to a greater or lesser degree. The greater the haemorrhage, the more the distension and the longer the recovery time, as the system has to break down and reabsorb the haemorrhage.

Anything that controls the haemorrhage naturally reduces the length of the recovery time.

There is a further danger. Further haemorrhage may occur if the athlete resumes competition too early. This can lead to ectopic calcification and myositis ossificans, or bony spur, that may interfere with quadriceps action.

There may be severe post-traumatic pain and hot swelling. It may be tender to touch, movement is limited (especially flexion), and the tenderness gets worse with time. Orthodox management of the condition mainly aims to limit the disability. Homoeopathic remedies will help effective healing.

Arnica
Taken in any potency immediately after the trauma, Arnica will limit the haemorrhage and greatly reduce the possibility of myositis ossificans traumatica.
Dosage: One Arnica 30c, immediately after the injury. Use Ruta, Rhus Tox. and Bryonia as necessary, according to the symptoms.

Hecla Lava
Has the power to arrest exostoses and bony growths that are sensitive and painful to touch.
Dosage: One Hecla Lava 200c daily for two weeks.

Rhus Toxicodendron
This remedy has a special affinity with bony outgrowths, and has been known to reduce them if the patient manifests other Rhus Tox. symptoms. It may prevent their development.
Dosage: One Rhus Tox. 200c daily for two weeks.

Quadriceps Strains

Treat strains of the quadriceps homoeopathically with Arnica, followed by the appropriate remedy. See those listed immediately above.

Groin Strain and Pain

Groin strain and pain are a common cause of layoffs among soccer, rugby and hockey players. The condition is difficult to diagnose and to manage. Fortunately you can prescribe homoeopathic medicines on the symptoms presented by the patient without long investigations. They will not interfere with any other treatment, have no side effects and will promote healing if correctly prescribed and used.

CASE 21

Peter, aged 40, is an international hockey player. He complained of paroxysmal cramping pain in the groin that seemed to come on when he was sitting at his desk, especially in the morning after a match. The pain was so violent it frightened him. He was very worried that it meant a hernia, and was afraid to cough in case it produced the condition. There was no record of trauma, and the condition had come on suddenly. He was reluctant to keep playing and his GP had advised against it, but offered no diagnosis.

A long case-taking gave me some insight into Peter's mental, emotional and general symptoms. He was very enthusiastic about everything, work, and play, and was a great organiser. He hated time-wasting in any form, and had to be busy all the time. He became bored very easily. He admitted drinking too much, quite often, but enjoyed alcohol. He sometimes felt very bad the morning after a party and avoided breakfast. He was irritable with people who should know their jobs. 'I get furious' was how he described his reactions. He often woke at about 3 a.m. and could not get back to sleep unless he made a list of all the things that occurred to him then about work. He hated cold windy days unless he could be active. Asked to sum up his approach to life he described himself as impatient for the next day.

Peter's mental and emotional symptoms were clearly those of Nux Vomica, but the remedy only has inguinal pain from coughing and 'as if he has a hernia'. I gave him Nux Vom. 10M, one at night for three nights.

One month later he reported that he had experienced no more episodes of pain and had continued playing hockey. He questioned whether my remedy could have affected the way he worked because he felt much calmer and positive. Three months later he was still free of pain. Six months later, still no pain, and he told me he had decided to take a redundancy scheme that would allow him to work at a more relaxed and much less stressful job.

Comment

The lesson from Peter's case is that the correctly chosen homoeopathic remedy will work despite the lack of an orthodox diagnosis. This is not to say that I do not always refer sports injury patients for diagnosis and orthodox treatment, but when one system does not satisfy the patient's needs, another may. I would always refer patients reporting inguinal or rectal pain for diagnosis, because of potential underlying pathology.

Some remedies that have inguinal pain among their more specific spheres of action are given below. However, the remedies are more likely to work if other symptoms match too. Choose one according to the manifested and detailed symptomatology.

Berberis

Aching tension in the groin, which is very painful to touch. Sensation that something will protrude when walking or standing. Throbbing, shooting pain in groin, extends to the testes and thighs and into the back. Worse from jarring and stepping hard, walks very tenderly and carefully. Groin pain may be associated with backache and urinary problems.

Dosage: One Berberis 30c hourly during the worst of the pain. Stop when the pain eases, then one daily for seven days.

Bryonia

Cramp-like, stitching, cutting and shooting pains in the groin, which is very tender. The pains come on even when sitting but are much worse from any movement, especially abduction of the leg.

Dosage: One Bryonia 30c hourly for three or four doses, then daily for up to seven days.

Calcarea Carbonica

The pains of Calc. Carb. are typically stitching, inguinal and the result of a sprain following physical exertion. The condition may follow exertion after the person has been warm and cooled off. This remedy has an affinity with the inguinal glands and could be effective if infection is a suspected cause of the pain. There may also be painful haemorrhoids that are worse when walking and better sitting. The person is typically slow-moving and indolent. You may think of them as flabby. Cold feet and hands.

Dosage: One Calc. Carb. 30c daily for three days.

Mercurius Solubilis

Cutting, stitching pains in the lower abdomen and groin, worse from walking. Sensation of knives in the groin. Painfully sensitive when walking or standing. Especially painful on the left side. The person is worse from being heated and from draughts, from sweating, and lying on the right side, tends to speak in hurried way and time passes very slowly for them.

Dosage: One Mercurius 30c, three times daily until the pain eases, but for not more than seven days.

Adductor Strain

This condition is sometimes called groin strain or rider's strain and comes about because of a tear in the adductor longus muscle when it is used for propulsion as in sprinting, lunging and twisting on a straight leg. It can be caused by sudden overstretching while sitting with the legs abducted, the dancer's 'second position'. It can be the cause of long-term indisposition.

Arnica
Dosage: One Arnica 30c or 200c immediately the pain occurs.

Ruta Graveolens
Dosage: One Ruta 30c or 200c three times daily during rehabilitation, but for not more than one month.

Bursitis

See under 'Bursae and Bursitis' in the knee section above (pages 126–8).

Bones and Fractures

CASE 22

A 35-year-old broke his femur in a climbing accident and had been lying on a ledge for three hours before being rescued. I saw him when he had been in hospital for four hours. A chest X-ray showed much effusion into his lungs, and he was in shock and hypothermic. Arnica 10M was indicated, and I gave him enough to take one tablet hourly for three doses.

He had been very cold and frightened and there was a lot of pain, which the Arnica relieved. I gave him Aconite for the fright and to help with the pain. His lungs cleared in two days, and there was little sign of the traumatic accident in the way of bruising.

He was to spend six weeks in traction. Bach Rescue Remedy and Aconite helped him to sleep and to relieve the pain. He took Symphytum 6c three times daily for the duration of his stay in hospital to promote bone formation and healing. He performed a rigorous daily programme of exercises, including isometrics for both legs and upper body strength.

A week after discharge he returned to work in a hinged full leg brace. He was able to exercise daily, but his ankle swelled badly after sitting.

First movement was painful. Continued movement relieved his pain and restlessness. Interferential treatment promoted healing and gave analgesia.

He took Rhus Tox. 30c as the symptoms demanded and used Bryonia 30c when he felt that movement would be painful. I gave him a stock of remedies and briefed him on their use, but he called me regularly to ask which one to take.

Ten weeks after his accident he was jogging lightly. Twelve weeks after it he was climbing again. Twelve years later he is still very fit and active. Helped by good orthotics he climbs, runs and exercises, and has recently completed a major expedition to the Himalayas.

Comment
This is only one of many cases I could quote of rapid healing of fractures and return to active sport as a result of homoeopathic treatment combined with physiotherapy.

All fractures need Arnica as a first remedy. Then, depending on the symptoms presented, a selection of remedies may be used. Symphytum promotes bone healing. Stress fractures of the femur will respond in the same way as described for those of the tibia.

Young People

One should always be conscious of the potentially serious implications of pain in the hip, femur and knee in young people. If you suspect a slipped femoral epiphysis, Perthes' disease or osteogenic sarcoma of the femur you should at once refer the patient for a medical diagnosis. Homoeopathy can help these conditions, but only when prescribed by a qualified homoeopath.

Nerve Pain

Tingling, numbness and pain may be felt down the front and lateral aspect of the thigh from pressure on the lateral head of the inguinal ligament. The pressure is usually from tight clothing or equipment and this must be removed or loosened. One Ruta 30c three times daily will help to relieve the discomfort.

Refer also to 'Sciatica', page 161.

GENITAL INJURIES

Male Genitalia

Injury to the genitalia is frequent in men, and they must be referred for medical attention. Male athletes should be encouraged to wear suitable protection for the scrotum and penis during competition and training. Traumatic injury to the scrotum may occur from contact with another athlete or dancer or equipment. The immediate result is usually incapacitating pain, and serious long-term effects may be precipitated.

Injury to the testicles may occur during and after cycling. The same remedies may be used according to the symptoms. Torsion of the testicles usually presents as a painful testicle and must be referred to a doctor.

Priapism, or persistent erection, caused by cycling may respond to Cantharis, but the patient should be referred to a doctor or a professional homoeopath.

Cold applications may help to relieve the pain but the following remedies will be more effective. Only give one at a time in the 6c potency:

Arnica

If given immediately, Arnica will relieve the pain, prevent haemorrhage, bruising and swelling, and encourage healing. If given later it will reduce swelling and bruising. The scrotum feels bruised and sore. The person may be in shock from the injury, but will say that he feels fine. He avoids further injury and touch.

Dosage: One Arnica 30c three times in one day will also reduce the possible development of haematorrhoea.

Bellis Perennis

This remedy has a special affinity with soft tissue injuries, and haemorrhages following blows to parts consisting of such sensitive tissue. The pains may be throbbing, aching or squeezing, and are so unbearable they drive him to distraction. He may have become chilled after being hot, and wants to keep moving to keep warm. He cannot bear touch, but is better from cold applications.

Dosage: One Bellis 30c for up to six doses, if Arnica has not relieved the pain and discomfort.

Cantharis

Painful, continuous erection with burning, smarting, cutting and raw pains with secretion of semen. Constant desire to urinate, but urine is passed only drop by drop. Excessive sexual desire. Blood in semen. Extremely hyperactive, not just sexually, with anxious restlessness. Shivering. Better from warmth and rest.

Dosage: One Cantharis 30c every twenty minutes for up to six doses, or until the condition eases if this is earlier.

Conium Maculatum

This remedy has the reputation for preventing serious repercussions from genital injury. It could be taken routinely after an injury.

Dosage: One Conium 200c daily for three days.

Euphrasia

The genitals retract spasmodically with a feeling of pressure above the pubic bone. Tingling pain in the testes. Sore, burning pain when touched. Lancinating pain in the glans penis.

Dosage: One Euphrasia 30c daily for three days.

Hypericum

Shooting pains in the genitals after a blow. The genitals are very painful and sore and very sensitive to touch, even from clothing. Movement is very painful, and he is afraid of jarring.

Dosage: One Hypericum 30c three times daily for three days.

Natrum Arsenicum

This remedy, if taken immediately after the injury, will relieve the feelings of nausea after a blow to the genitalia.

Dosage: One Natrum Arsenicum 30c should be sufficient.

Rhododendron

When the testes are swollen, painful, feel crushed, and are drawn up after injury. The scrotum may be inflamed. There is a drawing pain from the spermatic cord into the abdomen and thighs. Injury to the glans penis when that feels crushed. The pain may be tearing, and he feels paralysed. He feels worse in cold, wet windy weather.

Dosage: One Rhododendron 30c daily for three days.

Rhus Toxicodendron

The scrotum and penis become thick, swollen and oedematous. The pain is shooting, tearing and stitching, and is worse at night. He cannot find a comfortable position in which to sleep, and must keep changing position. First movement is painful. He is very restless, and has to move all the time because continued movement relieves the pain. The genital condition may have resulted from a blow, overlifting or overexertion.
Dosage: One Rhus Tox. 30c. Repeat if necessary.

Female Genitalia

Injury to the female genitalia may become more common with the increased popularity of soccer and rugby for women. Arnica is the first remedy to use for bruising. If bleeding from the vagina or labia occurs as a result of injury and has not been stopped by Arnica, one of the following remedies may be useful. It is imperative that if bleeding continues even a short time after the injury, the woman should see a doctor for assessment and treatment.

Female participants in long distance and stamina events who develop sore nipples will find that Calendula cream relieves this, and that Arnica or Causticum taken orally before the event helps to prevent the soreness becoming too painful.

Bellis Perennis

This remedy has a special affinity with soft tissue injuries and haemorrhages following blows to parts consisting of sensitive tissue. The pains may be throbbing, aching or squeezing, and are so unbearable they drive her to distraction. She may have become chilled after being hot, and wants to keep moving to keep warm. She cannot bear touch, but is better from cold applications.
Dosage: One Bellis 30c every few minutes for up to six doses if Arnica and Hamamelis have not stopped the bleeding.

Hamamelis

The vagina feels bruised and sore, tender, swollen and inflamed. There is bleeding, but she seems surprisingly unconcerned and tranquil about it. The abdomen may also be sore and feel bruised. She does not want to move, and prefers to keep warm and stay indoors. She does not want ice or cold applications.
Dosage: If Arnica has not stopped the bleeding, give Hamamelis 30c every fifteen minutes for six doses while awaiting medical attention.

SHOULDER INJURIES

The dominant shoulder is the most often damaged in sporting injuries. As right-handed players predominate in sports the right shoulder represents about 70% of the injuries to this region.

Pain in the shoulder may refer from the cervical spine, and it is vital to establish whether this is so. Everyone complaining of shoulder pain should be checked for a full range of painless movement in the neck. Checking the alignment of the head will sometimes help diagnosis.

From a homoeopathic point of view, pain originating in the neck and extending into the shoulder will be an important symptom that adds to the overall totality of symptoms that help choose the remedy. The correct remedy chosen according to that totality will naturally cure the neck problem too. I always refer such patients to an osteopath or chartered physiotherapist.

The following case demonstrates how a homoeopathic remedy can work at all levels. Even when the patient came about her sore throat, the remedy worked on her neck and shoulder, and may even have helped her to make up her mind about changing jobs.

CASE 23

Helen is a county standard lacrosse player who came to me about a persistent sore throat that made her hoarse and she also mentioned pain in her shoulder. She described the pain as 'rheumatic' because it seemed like the pain her mother also had. She described herself as a very sensitive person who always thought about other people's problems. She worked as a manager of a very busy town-centre coffee shop, but was planning a change of career because of the stress of business. She was planning to move into one of the caring professions, but could not make up her mind to move.

In my consulting room I noticed that her nose was about 30mm off the central line of her spine, and that her neck seemed stiff. I asked her about her neck, and she agreed it was so stiff it was difficult to move her head. I recommended an osteopath, and prescribed one Causticum 30c three times daily for three days.

The Causticum helped both her throat and her shoulder.

She telephoned me the day following her first osteopathic treatment because she was suffering sharp, cutting and intolerable pain in her neck in reaction to the treatment, and it was radiating into her shoulder. Her spine felt very sensitive, and movement made it worse.

Hypericum is a good remedy for pains in nerve-rich parts, and to follow injury, shock and concussion to the spine. It eases the pain in reaction to manipulative treatment, and Helen took one Hypericum 30c routinely after every treatment. In three months she had enrolled on a social work course, her throat, shoulder and neck were free of pain, and she was enjoying her lacrosse again.

Rotator Cuff and Tendons

The muscles that insert into the capsule of the glenohumeral joint combine in a sheet of tendon known as the rotator cuff. It reinforces the joint as well as enabling the muscles to act as stabilisers and movers. The rotator cuff is relatively easily injured by such actions as throwing or overhead racquet shots from an unusual arm or body position. An acute rotator cuff tear produces severe pain, weakness, bruising and can lead to swelling, limited mobility, pain and weakness.

The pain experienced is sometimes tearing, sore, neuralgic, or as if sprained or aching. Any movement of the arm or shoulder may be painful. Abduction, adduction, raising the arm and rotating the shoulder may be painful. There may be swelling, stiffness, weakness and perhaps a feeling of paralysis. Rest, relief of pain and restoration of a complete range of pain-free movements comprise the normal management of the injury. Choose a homoeopathic remedy that is appropriate to the symptoms, but begin with Arnica.

Arnica

A tear to part of the rotator cuff inevitably produces bleeding and its consequences. Arnica taken soon after the injury will help to reduce the pain, shock, bleeding, immobilisation and consequent recovery time.
Dosage: One Arnica 30c hourly for two days, reducing in frequency as symptoms improve. Repeat one dose if the pain returns.

Bryonia

The main symptom for Bryonia is that *any* movement is painful, and the person avoids it. The arm and shoulder feel too weak to move. Raising the arm is very painful and makes him feel bad. The joint feels swollen and hot. The pain is burning and tearing, and the shoulder feels pulled out of place. Pressure relieves the pain, so that he is most comfortable when lying on the injured shoulder. The pain is better from heat applied locally to the shoulder, but the patient feels worse from heat in general. The person feels discouraged, and averse to conversation.
Dosage: One Bryonia 30c.

Chelidonium

Painful right shoulder. Unable to use the arm. The least touch is exceedingly painful. Abduction is exceptionally painful. There is tearing, neuralgic and rheumatic pain. The arm feels heavy, stiff and flabby and there may be trembling. The pain may extend from the shoulder to under the scapula, and there may be a stiff neck. Although touch makes it worse, pressure may relieve the pain. Worse from any change of weather, from warmth, at 4 a.m. Restless, depressed and anxious, as if he had done something wrong. Chelidonium is similar to Bryonia in that movement is painful, but Chelidonium's stiffness is more rigid, and the muscles are more in spasm. Bryonia is afraid to move; Chelidonium cannot move.

Dosage: If Bryonia does not work on an injured right shoulder, try one Chelidonium 30c.

Ferrum Metallicum

Ferrum also affects the right shoulder, but when this remedy is indicated the person insists on trying to lift his arm even though it is extremely painful to do so. Moving the arm is intensely painful. You will notice this patient because he keeps trying to lift his arm gingerly to relieve the pain. There may be cracking or crepitus in the joint, and the pain may be tearing and stinging, and is worse at night. The person may be excitable, nervous and sensitive to the least noise. Feels much better when working or doing something.

Dosage: One Ferrum 30c if the symptoms fit.

Rhus Toxicodendron

This remedy may be useful at any time during recovery, especially if first movement is painful and continued movement relieves the pain. See Chapter 10 for details.

Dosage: One Rhus Tox. 30c daily for not more than two weeks.

Ruta Graveolens

Because of the damage to tendons, Ruta should be given regularly during recovery. The pains are sore, bruised, and aching and the arms are restless. See Chapter 10 for details.

Dosage: One Ruta 30c, daily for not more than two weeks.

Sanguinaria Canadensis

Cutting or stabbing pain felt in the right deltoid, worse on raising the arm. A feeling of rheumatism in the right shoulder. The shoulder pain is much worse at night and seems to be in the bones, especially the acromion and the greater tuberosity. Neuralgic pain which is relieved by touching the part. The pain may also be relieved by swinging the arm back and fore. The shoulder feels burning hot. He feels better from a good sleep, but may be morose and he grumbles about things.

Dosage: One Sanguinaria 30c.

CASE 24

While on a cross-country run, Robert vaulted over a gate. He described what happened next.

'I put my right hand on the gate and swung up. My right arm seemed to be supporting me, but suddenly it gave way. I fell from the top of my vault with a great heavy fall on my side. I was terribly shaken from the fall, but, worse of all, my right arm did not want to work any more. I could not lift it any way without a great deal of pain. I walked home slowly, and in pain.'

I saw him the next day. He was still in pain, feeling bruised all over, had not slept well, and wondered whether he should go to casualty. Strangely, though, as he walked in I asked him how he was and he said, 'Oh! I'm fine thanks.' I also noticed that he was very careful that no-one came anywhere near his arm and shoulder. One Arnica 30c three times a day for two days helped with the pain and discomfort. He was immediately less shocked, and agreed to see a physiotherapist colleague who diagnosed a partial tear in the rotator cuff.

Two days later Robert called me to say that his shoulder was very painful, and could I help? He had woken at 4 a.m. with intense pain and stiffness in his shoulder and neck. Any movement of his arm hurt badly. I gave him one Bryonia 30c. He called again later that evening to say he was still in pain. His neck was worse, the pain was spreading around his back and the only relief seemed to be a hot bath. He wondered if he had something more serious like a dislocation. His arm felt like a heavy dead weight. Abduction was the most painful movement. I gave him Chelidonium 30c to take whenever he had the pain.

Two weeks later he came to the clinic for physiotherapy and was feeling much better. He was still quite depressed and blaming himself for his injury. I gave him one Ruta 30c to take three times daily for a week to help his tendons recover.

Six weeks later he called again. He had played a hard game of squash, the first since his injury, and after one backhand shot felt a nasty twinge in his shoulder. This was a symptom caused by overexertion, and typical of Ruta. He took Ruta 200c, one tablet on waking, for two days.

Chronic Tendinitis

Chronic tendinitis tends to be more common among older sports people, and younger athletes and dancers who ignore the warning signs. It is often the result of overuse and repetitive stress of the joint. Although the actual site of the tendon affected may not be important for choosing the best homoeopathic remedy, the action which caused the injury may well be. For example, excessive repetitions of a weight training exercise such as a military press could be assessed as an injury caused by lifting, and you could choose a remedy which has lifting in its causation. Many chronic tendinitis conditions are caused by a throwing action. The nearest rubric we have to this in the homoeopathic repertory is 'Pain, sprained, as if'.

The problem with chronic tendinitis in the shoulder, from the patient's point of view, is that the pain limits his activity. Pain with movement is a constant reminder of the incapacity and this may make him despair of recovery. Some people are reluctant to take anti-inflammatory drugs continuously because of the side effects, and are even more reluctant to submit to steroid injections. The condition may therefore become incapacitating.

There are homoeopathic remedies which, in conjunction with physiotherapy, osteopathy and acupuncture, have been helpful in reducing pain and promoting healing. I have found that once a person begins to be able to move the shoulder and arm more freely, he becomes more positive about recovery. Rehabilitation exercises become more acceptable and the underlying distress of long-term injury can be alleviated.

Arnica
Although Arnica is more commonly associated with the immediate treatment of traumatic injury such as falls or blows, it is sometimes indicated if the shoulder feels sprained and the condition was brought on by overlifting and straining. For example, a weightlifter who increases his overhead press weight may gradually feel increasing pain in his shoulder. His shoulder is better when his arm hangs down. He complains of lack of strength in his hands when grasping something. He fears touch and further injury.

Dosage: Arnica 30c, once daily for as long as necessary to control the pain, but for not longer than two weeks. I sometimes find that a higher potency is more effective when the original pain was some time ago, and would give one dose of Arnica 200c as a first remedy in such a case. Repeat this if the pain returns.

Ferrum Metallicum
See page 141 above.
Dosage: It would be appropriate to use the 200c potency in cases of chronic tendinitis, one daily until relief is felt, but for not longer than two weeks.

Phosphorus
Tearing pain in the left shoulder, worse at night. Weakness in the affected arm on exertion, sometimes with trembling. The condition may have arisen from overlifting and overuse generally, and the onset will have been gradual. The joint may be stiff without pain. Sleeping on the left side makes it worse. Worse in the morning and evening, and when tired. This person likes to have his shoulder massaged, is very sensitive to the feelings of others and likes sympathy. The shoulder condition seems to come and go with the weather, day and night, wet and dry, etc. Often suitable for young dancers who have grown very quickly and have very flexible joints.
Dosage: Phosphorus 200c one daily in chronic cases. Stop the remedy when the condition begins to improve, but do not take for longer than two weeks.

Rhus Toxicodendron
This remedy is very specific for conditions brought on by overlifting, overstretching and overuse. See above for symptoms.
Dosage: Rhus Tox. 200c, one tablet. Repeat as necessary. Stop the remedy when the condition begins to improve, but do not take for longer than two weeks.

Ruta Graveolens
See Chapter 10 for symptoms.
Dosage: One Ruta 200c.

Sanicula
This remedy is indicated specifically when the pain is worse from putting the hands behind the back, and when raising the arms. The

condition will originate with strain, and will be worse from motion. The person may be headstrong, obstinate and irritable, and does not want to be touched.

Dosage: One Sanicula 200c daily. Stop the remedy when the condition begins to improve, but do not take for longer than two weeks.

Dislocation and Instability

A forced movement involving rotation and abduction, a fall on to an outstretched arm, or tackling in rugby can give rise to a common shoulder injury – that of dislocation. Both anterior and posterior dislocations cause considerable pain. Reduction of the joint may be achieved by skilled qualified staff soon after the injury, but delayed reduction after muscle spasm and inflammation has set in will be much more difficult. In any case there will be the likelihood of sequelae to the trauma. These can be helped by homoeopathic remedies in lessening the effects of the trauma and to promote healing of the capsule, rotator cuff and associated tissue.

If immediate reduction is proposed, it will be much more effective if the patient has received a dose of Arnica in any potency. This will enable the athlete or dancer to relax and be less fearful of the manipulation. It will also reduce the amount of haemorrhage from the tissues and the resultant inflammation, swelling, stiffness and incapacity. Arnica will also help to reduce the immediate pain. If reduction under anaesthetic is proposed, Arnica 30c, three doses the day before the operation, will speed recovery and reduce the possibility of complications.

If, following injury, the person is unwilling to move at all because of the pain, one Bryonia 30c hourly for five doses maximum will help.

CASE 25

A twenty-eight year old international rugby player suffered a subluxation of the right shoulder. It had been reduced immediately by the club physiotherapist. He still felt very shocked and in great pain. He had been operated on four years previously for the same problem in his left shoulder. As he still had pain in that shoulder he was very worried that he would have to have another operation. He denied that there as anything wrong with him 'apart from this stupid shoulder'. There was no point in going to see a doctor because he knew they could not help.

He was reluctant to be touched and winced if anyone came near. He slept very badly because of pain in the shoulder, but suggested it may have been because of a strange bed. The shoulder hurt less when he moved it, but if he carried on moving it became much worse.

Comment
He was given one dose of Arnica 1M immediately and the shoulder was gently massaged with Arnica oil. In this case Arnica fitted the patient's symptoms very closely, especially the denial of injury. He telephoned the next day to report that he felt 'much lighter', and that the swelling and pain in his shoulder was much reduced. A week later he was keen to begin training again. By the end of the same season he was back playing for the first XV, and scoring spectacular and robust tries.

Recovery Remedies
Other remedies will be useful during the recovery phase.

Causticum
There is a feeling of paralysis in the arm, and in the deltoid, so that he cannot raise his arm to his head. The pain is tearing, rheumatic and raw and is relieved by warmth, especially in bed. He tries to stretch, bend or crack his joints. He may describe the pain as if it feels dislocated or paralysed. There may be a cracking in the joints. You may have a feeling that without a lot of encouragement this patient is really going to have a paralysed shoulder. Anxious and depressed, very sensitive and guilty about being injured, he will feel that he has let down the team or the company.
Dosage: One Causticum 30c three times daily until improvement begins, or for a maximum of one week.

Rhus Toxicodendron
Tearing and burning sensation in the shoulder, worse when resting, and in bed. The right arm is weak and feels rheumatic. First movement is painful while continued movement relieves the pain. The person is very restless. Cannot rest in any position, and is inclined to keep moving. Worse at night, when cold, and when wet. Better after a hot bath. Rhus Tox. may be needed later in rehabilitation.
Dosage: One Rhus Tox. 30c taken last thing at night or first in the morning, for a week.

146

Ruta Graveolens

Wrenching pain in the shoulder that is worse when the arm hangs down (Arnica is better when the arm hangs down), and when resting on it. So he will be supporting his arm, which is typical of someone who has dislocated his shoulder. There will be a dull tearing pain in the humerus, and he feels bruised. The shoulder may be rigid, and later is very weak. Worse when cold, damp, sitting and lying. Because of the damage to tendons, Ruta should be given regularly during recovery. The pains are sore, bruised, and aching and the arms are restless.

Dosage: One Ruta 30c daily for two to three weeks maximum.

You may also give Ferrum, Phosphorus or Sanicula if the symptoms are appropriate. See the details above and in Chapter 10.

Frozen Shoulder

As the number of older people participating in active sport increases, the incidence of 'frozen shoulder' or 'adhesive capsulitis' becomes more frequent. It is uncertain whether this is because sports involve a wider range of shoulder movements, and the sports person notices the limitation earlier, or that more sports participation to a greater age predisposes the sufferer to injury. Whatever the cause, movement at the shoulder becomes limited, either by pain or stiffness, and the person complains that the normal activities of living become difficult.

Joint mobilising techniques may be the preferred treatment, and can resolve the condition. Unfortunately, this condition can easily become permanent, with the shoulder self-limiting to a very small range of movements. I see too many older patients who have not been able to lift their arms for months or even years, and who still expect miracles. I usually treat them constitutionally, that is with the remedy that fits their whole symptom picture.

Referral to an osteopath or chiropractor may help when the shoulder condition is generated by a problem in the region of the cervical spine. I have also known acupuncture to help. The normal expectation would be for the amount of mobility to improve over a period of eighteen months to two years, and for pain to diminish over the first six months. Homoeopathic medicines can help to relieve the pain.

CASE 26

Georgia is a high-powered executive in the public relations business. She likes to play golf and walk in the hills, and at the age of fifty still considers herself very fit. Her osteopath suggested she should come to see me because her right shoulder had become very stiff, her voice was very hoarse and she felt under too much stress at work.

She could not raise her arm above shoulder height, and even that was with an extreme lifting of the shoulder girdle. The pain was awful every morning and made her scream. She slept with her arm under her head, but that made her shoulder extremely painful and stiff. She had had rheumatoid arthritis as a child, and it now seemed to be settled in her shoulder. It hurt to move it. The pain made her weep, and she cried as she told me about it.

The stress at work came from her feeling that neither her clients nor her bosses appreciated her. She worked hard, but was indignant that she did not get the recognition she deserved. If someone criticised her she felt 'really awful. I could scream, but I keep it inside'.

She talked about her husband who had died three years earlier, and said that she had never really grieved for him at the time. Now the grief was with her all the time.

Georgia's remedy was Staphysagria. I gave her the 200c potency because of the balance of mental, emotional and physical symptoms; indignation, bottling up her emotions, anger especially, feeling unappreciated, her unresolved grief, sensitivity to criticism, intolerable tearing pain in shoulder and hoarseness.

She took one tablet morning and night for three days. Her voice was better at once. She felt better about work and was less stressed. With prolonged mobilising and manipulation her shoulder improved gradually, and six months later she had 70% mobility.

Although I would recommend that someone like Georgia who had a chronically frozen shoulder should see a specialist or a qualified homoeopath for an in-depth consultation, there are a few remedies that could help in the short term.

Bryonia
This may be useful if the slightest movement is painful.
Dosage: One Bryonia 30c. Repeat as necessary for up to seven days.

Ferrum Metallicum
Ferrum may be effective for a frozen right shoulder. The person insists on trying to lift his arm even though it is extremely painful to do so. Moving the arm is intensely painful. There may be cracking or crepitus in the joint, and the pain is tearing and stinging. It is worse at night.

Look for an excitable, nervous person who is sensitive to the least noise. He feels much better when working or doing something.
Dosage: One Ferrum 200c three times daily if the symptoms fit, for not more than seven days.

Lycopodium

The condition may have originated with lifting a weight and begun as a stiff neck. Tearing and shooting pain in the right shoulder, with tension and weakness. It feels as if arthritis were attacking the shoulder, and this makes it difficult to move the arm. The pain is worse at night, and on waking from sleep. It may be worse at about 4 p.m. Tends to keep moving his arm to relieve the pain.
Dosage. One Lycopodium 30c daily until the pain is relieved, then take one as necessary, for not more than seven days.

Natrum Muriaticum

A paralytic heaviness of the arm with a wrenching pain in the shoulder prevents the arm from being moved or elevated. The shoulder feels sprained. There may also be aching and rigidity in the neck with painful stiffness. Trembling of the hands may accompany the shoulder symptoms. The pain is worse between 9 a.m. and 11 a.m. and may come on then. This person dislikes the heat of the sun. She cannot stand sympathy and brushes it off or ignores it.
Dosage: One Natrum Mur. 200c three times daily, for not more than seven days.

Rhus Toxicodendron

Burning pains in the shoulder with stiffness brought on by overexertion or lifting a weight. The right arm feels weak and paralysed, especially at night and in bed or at rest. Stiffness and pain are worse on first movement but relieved by constant motion. The patient is restless and always moving. There is painful tension of the neck when he tries to move his arm, but this eases with movement.
Dosage: One Rhus Tox. 200c taken last thing at night or first in the morning as necessary, for not more than seven days.

Ruta Graveolens

Wrenching pain in the shoulder that is worse when the arm hangs down, and when resting on the arms. Neck symptoms probably absent. There will be a dull tearing pain in the humerus, and he feels bruised. The shoulder is rigid, and very weak. He feels worse when cold, damp, sitting and lying. He may be anxious, nervous, restless and depressed in the late evening. Because of the damage to tendons, Ruta should be given regularly during recovery. The pains are sore, bruised, and aching and the arms are restless.

Dosage: One Ruta 200c daily for two to three weeks.

Acromioclavicular Sprain

Falling on to the point of the shoulder is a common cause of damage in the acromioclavicular joint among rugby lock forwards, horse riders and cyclists, as well as mountain bikers who fall and land on their shoulder. There may be some tearing in the acromioclavicular and coracoclavicular ligaments which normally stabilise the joint, and there may be springing of the lateral end of the clavicle. There is tenderness, pain and swelling over the top of the shoulder and pain when the scapula moves. The pain can go on for three to six weeks.

Arnica
This remedy is very specific for injuries from a fall. Take it immediately after the fall and every hour for the remainder of day. It will prevent shock, relieve the immediate pain and reduce the internal damage, haemorrhage, inflammation and swelling.

Dosage: One dose of Arnica taken immediately in any potency will help.

Bryonia
If any movement is painful following injury Bryonia will make it easier.

Dosage: One Bryonia 30c for not more than six doses.

Chelidonium
See page 00 above.

Dosage: If Bryonia does not work on an injured right shoulder, try Chelidonium 30c three times daily, for not more than seven days.

Rhus Toxicodendron
See above and Chapter 10.

Ruta Graveolens
Helps to promote healing of ligaments and tendons.

Dosage: One Ruta 30c three times daily, for not more than seven days.

Sanguinaria

He cannot raise or rotate the right arm. Movement makes it really much worse, especially moving in bed. It is much worse at night in bed. Pain on top of the shoulder, in the acromioclavicular region, and in the deltoid. Rheumatic pain in the shoulder extending to the elbow. Pain under the scapula, worse moving and breathing. He may be irritable and morose, and unwilling to make any effort.

Dosage: One Sanguinaria 30c for not more than seven days.

CASE 27

A twenty-eight year old paralympic athlete who specialised in swimming and table tennis suffered terrible pains in his right shoulder and both wrists. The pain was worse during training on the road in wet weather, and was much better when training in the USA. His muscles were generally stiff and painful after sleep or sitting for long periods. He felt as if he had a hangover even if he had not been drinking. His head felt heavy. His arms were numb. His thirst for cold drinks was increased. The pains stopped him getting to sleep.

This person is restless, and finds it difficult to sit still for long. He is very impatient, and quite angry that his symptoms have stopped him training. Because he is recognised as being a successful athlete it gives him a sense of belonging to society despite his paralysis.

Comment

Because of his restlessness, continually changing position, worse in wet weather, better in warm sunny weather, impatience and anger at being injured, he was given Rhus Tox. 1M, one tablet. Ten minutes later he said that he felt strangely peaceful.

He was asked to report again the next day by telephone, but did not. A week later he rang to apologise for not telephoning. He had gone off on a training camp and had forgotten his condition.

ARM, ELBOW, WRIST AND HAND

Intramuscular Haematoma

Intramuscular haematoma of the biceps or triceps results from a blow to the upper arm in contact sports or cricket. The biceps will have become engorged with blood before and during a match and a blow ruptures blood vessels, causing a massive extravasation of blood.

Anything that controls the haemorrhage naturally reduces the length of the recovery time.

There is a further danger. If competition is resumed too early, there may be further haemorrhage. This can lead to ectopic calcification and myositis ossificans. The resultant bony spur may interfere with biceps action.

There may be severe post-traumatic pain and hot swelling. It may be tender to touch, flexion is limited, and the tenderness gets worse with time. Orthodox management of the condition aims to limit the disability. Homoeopathic remedies may be able to help.

Arnica
Arnica in any potency, taken immediately after the trauma, will limit the haemorrhage and greatly reduce the possibility of myositis ossificans traumatica.
Dosage: One Arnica 30c as soon as possible after the injury.

Bellis Perennis
Use this remedy if Arnica does not seem to work for bruising to soft tissue.
Dosage: One Bellis 30c.

Bryonia
If any movement is painful.
Dosage: One Bryonia 30c daily, repeated as necessary for up to seven days.

Hecla Lava
Hecla Lava has the power to arrest exostoses and bony growths that are sensitive and painful to touch.
Dosage: One Hecla Lava 200c daily for two weeks.

Rhus Toxicodendron

Rhus Tox. has a special affinity with bony outgrowths and has been known to reduce them if the patient manifests other Rhus Tox. symptoms (see Chapter 10).

Dosage: One Rhus Tox. 200c potency, one daily for two weeks.

Use Ruta, Rhus Tox. and Bryonia as necessary. Bryonia will be best if any movement is painful.

Lateral Epicondylitis (Tennis Elbow)

Although this is a common overuse injury in tennis and other racquet sports it is not confined to these alone, or indeed to sport at all. Any activity involving recurrent forced extension of the wrist or a sudden resisted movement will apply stress that tears muscle fibres from their origin in the lateral epicondyle of the humerus. If the stress is repeated before healing is complete the small scars will tear again, causing local bleeding and inflammation. Further repetition leads to the buildup of chronic inflammation.

The pain may be continuous and severe, and felt in the elbow as a burning or tearing. The pain often extends up or down the arm, or both. It may only be a twinge felt when gripping something or extending the wrist. It may prevent the person from gripping anything, or force them to drop things.

Orthodox management insists that rest from painful activity is essential, and that the arm should be kept in a sling if only to remind the patient not to use it. Physiotherapy with stretching, ice, contrast baths and splints may also be recommended. Orthodox treatment also recommends anti-inflammatory drugs, steroid injections for the pain and inflammation, and possibly surgery. I believe that homoeopathic remedies can be effective in relieving this condition. Their use could shorten recovery and healing time significantly.

Ideally the person should begin treatment immediately the pain starts, but the temptation is to 'work through the pain'. This is a recipe for chronic problems.

Golfer's Elbow (medial epicondylitis) presents similarly and could also respond to the following remedies.

Arnica

I would educate susceptible professional racquet players and golfers to take Arnica before every match, and especially later on in tough matches or tournaments. Arnica is a great preventative for intense over-use injury. Not only would it help to prevent tennis elbow, but would also help to reduce fatigue. I would add one Arnica 6c to the player's inter-set or game drink. If Arnica 30c is taken when the pain first appears, and repeated hourly, it will limit the damage and ease the pain. It will prevent inflammation and will avoid the need for hydrocortisone injections.

The specific symptoms for Arnica in this kind of injury are that there is weakness in the fingers when trying to grasp an object. There is pain in the arm, so that the person must allow it to hang down to relieve it. The person will say he feels fine, does not want any fuss or treatment that involves touching his elbow, and prefers to lie quietly somewhere. *Dosage:* One Arnica 30c, 200c or 1M, depending on the length of time since the condition first manifested, three times daily for two or three days.

Lachesis

This remedy is specifically effective for left elbows and hands when there is great weakness after overexertion. The condition comes on suddenly when the athlete or dancer wakes in the morning. It may come on every two weeks. There is pain in the elbow. The left arm is numb and weak, and there may be tingling in the left hand. The person feels generally weak. Look out for someone who tends to talk a lot about many subjects, and who may show signs of jealousy. Movement makes it worse.

Dosage: One Lachesis 30c or 200c three times daily for as long as necessary to control the pain, for a maximum of seven days.

Natrum Sulphuricum

The pain is in either elbow but extends to the hand, which feels weak. The player cannot grasp the racquet without pain. The pain is piercing, and the more he thinks about it the worse it becomes. This person is generally worse in damp weather and at night. Pressure and touch make the pain worse.

Dosage: One Natrum Sulph. 30c or 200c three times daily until relief, but for not longer than four weeks.

Rhus Toxicodendron

Rhus Tox. will help this condition if the pain is worse when resting, and on first movement, but where continued movement relieves it. The player moves his arm constantly. The pain is in either elbow, is paralysing and makes him nauseous. It centres in the humeral epicondyle. The elbow is hot, swollen and painful. The arm feels shaky.

Dosage: One Rhus Tox. 30c three times daily, or as often as necessary for the pain. Be sure to stop the remedy when the condition eases. If no relief is felt after five or six doses, change to another remedy.

Ruta Graveolens

As with every condition involving ligaments and tendons, Ruta can prove useful to help recovery, especially when the condition is the result of overexertion. Pain in the ulna and humerus. Stiffness extends to the wrist, and the fingers may contract.

Dosage: I have found that the most effective treatment protocol in this and similar tendon injuries is to give Ruta 30c three times daily for fourteen days, stop for fourteen days, and then repeat for another fourteen days if still necessary.

Dislocation of the Elbow

The recent popularity of relatively new sports such as cross country cycling, skateboarding and rollerblading have increased the incidence of elbow dislocations and traumatic damage. The traditional sports of riding, skiing, and gymnastics were more commonly the cause of this condition. Reduction is usually effective if undertaken immediately.

Arnica

A dose of Arnica 30c before reduction is attempted will make the athlete more likely to cooperate. The remedy will also make the athlete more amenable to early mobilisation of the joint. If reduction is conducted later under analgesia the athlete should take Arnica before and after the operation to reduce internal damage and shock and to promote recovery.

Dosage: One Arnica 30c before reduction is attempted. Then hourly for the first few hours, then three times daily for three days.

Bryonia

If any movement is painful Bryonia 30c will help make motion less painful.

Dosage: One Bryonia 30c for up to seven days.

Ruta Graveolens

Take this remedy for the tendon and ligament damage.

Dosage: I have found that the most effective treatment protocol in this and similar tendon injuries is to give Ruta 30c three times daily for fourteen days, stop for fourteen days, and then repeat for another fourteen days if still necessary.

Tenosynovitis of the Wrist and Forearm

Oral NSAIDs and injected steroids are often bought over the counter or prescribed for tenosynovitis in the extensor tendons of the wrist. Gripping and grasping with extension of the wrist often induces this kind of tenosynovitis. Its symptoms often fit the remedy Rhus Tox., as in the following case.

CASE 28

Judy is a rock climber, aged 26. She complained of an intermittent pain medially in her right elbow and wrist. This was worse after a session on the climbing wall. Sometimes it prevented her training. The onset had been insidious and gradual.

She described the pain in her wrist as aching. It usually came on at night, and sometimes woke her after she had been lying on her arm. I noticed that as she told me about it she constantly moved her arm and wrist. The stiffness was, she said, worse when she got up in the morning, whether she had been on the climbing wall or not. When she had 'got it going' it improved and did not bother her. She felt that her hand was getting weak. She was worried that a climbing trip she had planned would have to be cancelled. She was due to leave in three weeks' time.

I gave her one Rhus Tox. 200c to take three times daily for three days, and advised her to stop training and to consult a physiotherapist colleague, who later diagnosed medial epicondylitis. He prescribed ultrasound and confirmed the need to rest.

She reported after a week to the effect that she felt much better. Her arm was not painful in the morning and she wanted to start climbing again. I advised against it. The improvement continued well enough for her to take the trip and enjoy it.

Tenosynovitis produces pain, weakness and stiffness in the wrist and hand. Frequently synovitis arises in the tendon of the extensor carpi radialis longus and of the pollicis muscles. It can also arise in the

156

tendons running through the carpal tunnel, and result in carpal tunnel syndrome.

From a homoeopathic point of view one takes the symptoms as they are described or observed, and chooses a remedy that fits those symptoms. Fortunately only a few remedies cover the common symptomatology of conditions affecting the tendons of the forearm and wrist.

Plumbum Metallicum

This remedy, derived from lead, will be useful when there is painful weakness of the wrist and hand. The wrist feels paralysed and may be dropped. There is difficulty in grasping objects. The symptoms appear very slowly and insidiously. There may be a sensation of a string pulling the wrist into extension or flexion. There may also be violent contraction of the fingers. The person definitely avoids being touched because it hurts. He may also avoid exertion, but likes massage because it makes him feel better. He may be a taciturn sort of person who is not keen on company.

Dosage: One Plumbum 30c daily for pain during recovery, for not more than two weeks.

Rhododendron

The wrist feels bruised and sprained. The pain is tearing, and there is a sensation of boring. There is stiffness, paralysis and weakness in the wrist and hand. The pain is worse at night and at rest. Unlike Rhus Tox., which is painful on first movement, Rhododendron is better as soon as movement begins. The person who needs Rhododendron will dislike storms and rough, windy weather. He will enjoy the sun.

Dosage: One Rhododendron 30c daily during recovery, for not more than a month.

Rhus Toxicodendron

Rhus Tox. will help this condition is the pain if worse when resting and on first movement, but relieved by continued movement. The player moves his arm, wrist and hand constantly. The pain can be in either wrist, is tearing, shooting and stitching and makes him nauseous. The wrist and hand are stiff and weak. His hand feels shaky. He is worse from exposure to cold and wet, and at night, and better from heat.

Dosage: One Rhus Tox. 30c daily as often as necessary for the pain. Be sure to stop the remedy when the condition eases.

Ruta Graveolens

Wrenching pain in the wrist that is worse when the arm hangs down, and when resting on them. There will be a dull tearing pain in the wrist, which feels bruised. The wrist may be rigid, and the hand very weak. He feels worse when cold, damp, sitting and lying. He may be anxious, nervous, restless and depressed in the late evening. Because of the damage to tendons Ruta should be given regularly during recovery. The pains are sore, bruised and aching and the arms are restless.

Dosage: One Ruta 200c daily for two weeks.

Sprains, Fractures and Dislocation of the Wrist

When someone talks of a sprained wrist he is usually describing an area of pain resulting from a traumatic incident. There may be a genuine sprain of the intercarpal ligaments with localised pain on passive flexion. A fall onto an outstretched hand may cause the condition, and can also produce a dislocation of a carpal bone or of the lunate. More important, there may be a fracture of the scaphoid. This again is associated with a fall onto the outstretched hand, as is the Colles's fracture in older sports persons and dancers.

Obviously, when someone presents with a history of a fall onto an outstretched hand, followed by intense pain in the wrist, correct specialist diagnosis is essential. Fractures to the scaphoid only heal with difficulty, and the practitioner needs to be sure that the correct diagnosis has been made.

Arnica

This remedy should be given automatically if the injury follows a fall.
Dosage: Immediately after the fall, one Arnica 6c. Between two days and a month after the fall, give Arnica 200c, three doses in one day. If the accident took place more than a month before the referral, give one dose of Arnica 1M.

Symphytum

This remedy will assist bone fusion if non-union is evident, especially for a fractured scaphoid and in painful old injuries.
Dosage: One Symphytum 30c.

Rhododendron, Rhus Tox. and Ruta may also be needed during recovery. See Ruta Graveolens above for prescribing protocol.

Injuries to Fingers

Cricketers and hockey players frequently suffer blows to and fractures of the phalanges from blows by the ball. They are very painful and often disabling. They normally require taping and gentle mobilising for three to four weeks. If the players were to take the following remedies they would avoid much of the pain, discomfort and layoff. Dislocations sometimes occur as the result of blows and falls, and should be reduced immediately if possible.

Arnica
Take it as soon as the injury occurs.
Dosage: One Arnica 30c as soon as possible.

Hypericum
Violent, shooting, piercing pain and soreness in nerve-rich parts always respond to Hypericum. The fingers are very sensitive to touch and jarring. The finger is much more painful than it appears and is better from rubbing. The player tends to rub it whenever possible.
Dosage: Hypericum 30c as frequently as necessary for the pain, for not more than ten doses.

Symphytum
This remedy will assist bone fusion, especially in painful old injuries.
Dosage: Symphytum 30c three times daily for two to three weeks.

Tendon and Ligament Injuries

The increasing popularity of skiing on artificial slopes has produced a spate of thumb injuries. These can be fractures or dislocations that should be given the same treatment as fractured fingers, ligament damage or rupture. Take Arnica immediately after the injury and repeat as necessary, followed by Hypericum if there is intense pain, and Symphytum to promote healing. Ruta will help ligaments to heal.

Mallet and buttonhole deformity injuries result from damage to the extensor tendon mechanism. They may require surgery or splinting. If they arise from trauma, Arnica is the first remedy to take. Following Arnica, Ruta can assist the tendons to heal.

Carpal Tunnel Syndrome

This condition is the result of compression of the median nerve as it passes beneath the transverse carpal ligament. The compression may be caused by inflammation and swelling of the tendons sharing the compartment, and may be the result of overuse. Gymnasts, cyclists, weightlifters and rock climbers, and any other sports persons habitually using hard gripping actions, may tend to overstrain the grip. Rock climbers work hard at achieving 'pump out' of the forearms, and this can contribute to inflammation of the tendons.

Although inflammation may not be the first indication, numbness, tingling and burning is felt in the fingers. The pain increases with movement. It typically wakes the sufferer at night. Hanging the hand down over the edge of the bed or shaking the hand relieves the 'pins and needles'.

Alumina
This remedy has the unusual symptom that the person feels as if a red hot needle is being inserted into the finger. The fingers are heavy, as if paralysed, with pins and needles after going to sleep. Wakes from the pain which is worse in bed. Loss of coordination. Worse in a warm room and after a warm bath. The condition may resolve without reason, and then later return. A hasty person for whom time passes too slowly. Grumpy on waking.
Dosage: One Alumina 30c three times daily for up to two weeks.

Apis Mellifica
Numbness of tips of fingers. Stinging pains that come on extremely suddenly. Feels as if stung by bee or wasp. Burning and soreness are present. The fingers may be red, swollen and itching. They are worse from touch of bedclothes and warmth of bed. He wants to keep cool, and hates heat. Awkward, and drops things. As with Arnica, he says there is nothing wrong and is indifferent to his condition.
Dosage: One Apis 30c three times daily for up to two weeks.

Arsenicum Album
Burning pain that is better from heat is a strange symptom and is peculiar to Arsenicum. The burning is like fire, hot needles or wires, and is maddening. He feels the pain when asleep, and it wakes him at about 2 a.m. It also has tingling in the fingers, which cannot be extended. The

hands tremble and twitch. They are suddenly very weak. The pains come on every two weeks, or with similar regularity. They are worse from cold and damp, and better from heat. The person has to walk about shaking the hand because of the pain, and is very restless. Careful with money and security. Very sensitive to things being in their correct place, and likes order. Set routines.

Dosage: Arsenicum 30c three times daily for up to two weeks.

Bryonia

Pins and needles in the fingers, following numbness. There is stitching pain with hot red swelling around the finger joints. The person does not want to move the fingers. He is better from pressure on the hand and likes to have it bound up tightly and kept cool. The hand is weak and cannot grip. He does not like being hot.

Dosage: One Bryonia 30c three times daily for up to two weeks.

Calcarea Carbonica

Tearing, neuralgic pain in the fingers. Cold damp hands. Fingers are numb when gripping, and are stiff and immobile. Cramps at night, arthritic pain, and swelling. Worse from cold air, bathing and exertion, and may be depressed and sad about the condition. Weak wrists that sprain easily in heavily built, overweight, flabby, fair children, young people and adults. Worse from exertion, forgetful. Sweats about the head. Check on the typical Calc. Carb. type in the materia medica in Chapter 12.

Dosage: One Calc. Carb. 30c three times daily for up to two weeks..

Kali Carbonicum

There is a burning in the fingers that the person may describe as 'like fire'. The fingers are weak and numb, and the finger tips are very sensitive and painful with sharp stitching pains. These are worse after exertion and movement. The palm may also be very sensitive, and the arm jerks when it is touched. This chilly person wakes from the pain in the early morning, about 2–3 a.m., often from lying on the hand. Hyper-sensitive to pain, noise, draughts and touch; never contented or quiet. Argumentative and quarrelsome.

Dosage: One Kali Carb. 30c or 200c three times daily. Repeat the remedy as necessary, for up to two weeks.

Natrum Muriaticum
Numbness and tingling in the fingers with trembling of the hands when writing or performing delicate tasks. Cracks in the finger tips. A reserved and detached person who rarely cries or shows emotion and hates sympathy.
Dosage: One Natrum Mur. 30c daily for up to two weeks.

THE BACK AND NECK

Back pain affects millions of people. It is not limited to sedentary people and has significant effects on athletes and dancers. Individuals in these sectors of the community have strong incentives to return to activity, despite the pain.

It is important, therefore, for the athlete or dancer to receive a skilled diagnosis that will rule out tumour, infection, acute fracture, progressive neurological deficit, visceral sources and rheumatoid variants (Dreisinger and Nelson). When this has been done, a homoeopathic remedy prescribed according to the symptomatology can be effective in treating any condition.

Lower Back Pain
Although lower back conditions account for only a small number of sports injuries, the anatomical region accounts for a much larger part of the physiotherapist's, osteopath's and chiropractor's practice. The lower back is the most common site of injury in dancers. *Fit to Dance* quotes figures of 45% of the 658 dancers surveyed as suffering lower back injuries.

It is the single largest reason for loss of work in Britain and in Europe. Could it be that sports injuries have something to do with this? Or is it merely due to bad posture and incorrect function? Hard surfaces, raked stages, reluctance to eat, insufficient warm-up and low general fitness levels may also contribute to lower back injuries in dancers. Most of the presenting conditions are due to mechanical problems in the lumbar spine, which could be the result of long-forgotten trauma to the back or a long build up of stress.

Pain after exertion, standing, sitting or lying for a time is common. If it is eased by further exercise it is probably due to strain of the intra-vertebral and other supporting ligaments in the spine. The energy absorption qualities of these ligaments reduces with age. Advice on

162

improving technique, postural improvement, graduated exercises and careful stretching and correct warming up and down is appropriate.

Leg asymmetry can cause symptoms similar to ligamentous pain. Such asymmetry can be produced in dancers by frequent performance on raked stages, and in distance runners who regularly run on the same side of a cambered road or always in the same direction around a running track. Gymnasts, dancers, divers and other sports persons requiring hypermobility of the lumbar spine may also develop lower back pain. Overstretching should be avoided, and strengthening exercises are as important as mobilising.

Muscular Imbalance in Dancers

It is almost inevitable that dancers, especially ballet dancers, overwork some muscles while underworking others. The turnout required for ballet demands enhanced outward rotation of the hip, which can cause an imbalance in it. The quadriceps tend to become well developed, whereas the abdominals are often neglected. Strong trunk muscles lead to lumbar stability and better postural alignment. Traditional dance training concentrates on the limbs and head while neglecting the trunk. Dancers commonly have weak abdominal and lower back muscles, and this weakness can lead to lower back injury.

Orthodox Treatment

Orthodox treatment includes reducing activity in order to protect the body from further injury. This is often difficult in professional athletes, and more so among dancers. Avoiding painful positions and movements will help, as will ice and compression. Pain relief can be achieved with ice, ultrasound, manipulation, non-steroidal anti-inflammatory drugs and homoeopathic remedies. The latter can facilitate the body's own healing properties while the athlete or dancer undertakes proper exercise, stretching and light resistance exercises.

Homoeopathic Remedies

If the cause is obvious, always advise the person to eliminate it. There are homoeopathic remedies that can help by treating the presenting symptoms. Even these will not be effective if the maintaining cause is not eliminated.

Many of the following remedies have similar physical symptoms. When that is the case it makes choosing the correct one difficult. You must then rely on differentiating between remedies by using the mental and general symptoms that are peculiar to one of the remedies.

As a general rule, no remedy should be taken for more than, say, two weeks and should be discontinued earlier if relief is felt, as indicated below. The first remedy listed, Rhus Tox., has proved effective in relieving the pain in many cases and is a good standby.

Rhus Toxicodendron

The typical physical symptoms of lower back pain fit Rhus Tox. almost exactly, and I would expect it to eliminate pain in most cases. There is pain following exertion. Rest, sitting and lying aggravate the pain, and movement ameliorates it. Heat and hot bathing ameliorate. The pain is a contractive ache, and the back feels as if it would break on first moving. Hard pressure eases it. At rest and at night the pain radiates down the thigh. He is worse when the weather is wet and at night. He has disturbed nights, and dreams of great exertion. He should take Rhus Tox. 30c as necessary.

Dosage: One Rhus Tox. 30c before rest. Repeat as necessary, but for not more than two weeks.

Agaricus

The pain typically arises from fatigue. There is painful weakness and soreness in the lumbar region and sacrum with a sort of crick in the back. It is worse on stooping. The lumbar region feels dislocated, and worse when sitting or lying. The pain is increased by walking about or standing. (Rhus Tox. is relieved by walking about.)

Worse in the open air. The ligaments and muscles feel tight. Some spasm may be evident on palpation. The person feels worse in the morning and dislikes cold. He talks nervously, talks a lot, and is often quite funny.

Dosage: One Agaricus 30c three times daily until the pain eases, but for not more than two weeks.

Berberis

Backache with severe prostration and crushing, stitching, paralysing pain in lumbar region. Worse sitting and lying. It is also worse from standing and motion. The pain radiates down the front of the thighs. It is aggravated by rising from a seat. This person is very sensitive to jarring, and will complain if someone walks heavily or slams a door. Unwilling to walk even a short distance, because it makes him very tired.

Dosage: One Berberis 30c, as often as necessary for the pain, but for not more than two weeks.

Bryonia

Stitching pain in the small of the back that is worse from any movement. The pain is worse from turning and walking. Stiffness also prevents stooping. Any movement, even the least of any part makes this person feel bad. He may be frightened to move, to talk, or even to breathe because of the possibility of pain.

Dosage: One Bryonia 30c until the pain eases, but for not more than two weeks.

Lycopodium

Pain in lumbar region worse sitting, and worse motion. The person may need this remedy after Bryonia has eased the initial pain.

Dosage: One Lycopodium 30c as necessary for the pain, but for not more than two weeks.

Natrum Muriaticum

Almost the opposite of Rhus Tox., Natrum Mur. cannot straighten the back but can stoop easily. Paralysis in the lumbar region with painful stiffness. The spine is very sensitive. Tearing pains pulsate across the sacroiliac and into the hips. Tension and pulling in back. Bruised backache, worse early in the morning and again between 10 and 11 a.m. It hurts to cough, and is better when lying on the back on something hard. This person is worse from heat but enjoys massage. Hates sympathy.

Dosage: One Natrum Mur. 30c three times daily, but for not more than two weeks.

Sulphur

Lumbar pains following strenuous exertion such as a very hard game or run. The pain makes him walk bent. Can only straighten up after moving gently and stretching. He has to support himself on his hands when sitting. He has pain in his back when urinating. The least pressure on his back causes pain. Worse in bed, standing, and at 11 a.m. He is rather an untidy person, a bit of a dreamer and philosopher.

Dosage: One Sulphur 30c three times daily to relieve the pain, but for not more than two weeks.

Sacroiliac Injuries

Sacroiliac strains can be caused by actions that stress the joint during extension of the legs. A footballer at full stretch for a kick loses grip with his supporting foot, a fast bowler slips during delivery or a golfer with habitual bad posture disrupts the joint during a swing. A rugby prop forward puts enormous strain on his lower back during the collapse of a scrum.

Pain is mainly felt in the lower back, and may be located in the dimples of the sacrum. Sitting is usually comfortable. The pain is worst when standing up from a seat, bending backwards and twisting. It may also be painful when sitting. Pain may be referred down the back of the thigh and often gives the sensation of a shortened or strained hamstring. It may become worse at work for an athlete whose job involves bending over a desk or table.

There are several remedies that are almost specific for injuries to the sacrum as caused by blows, falls, overexertion and overstretching. Choose one to follow Arnica according to the symptoms. If the first choice does not relieve the pain in a few hours, try another.

Arnica
This is the first remedy to take whenever there has been traumatic injury such as a strain, fall, twist, blow or slip.
Dosage: One Arnica 30c immediately after the injury, and repeat as often as necessary for the first few hours, or for not more than six doses.

The following may also be of use:

Aesculus Hippocastanum
Constant ache in the sacrum that is much worse from bending forward and walking. It is almost impossible to rise after sitting. The sacrum feels bruised and weak. The pain may strike suddenly, and prevents him from working or training. Worse on waking in the morning. He is very irritable.
Dosage: One Aesculus 30c three times daily until the pain is relieved, or for not more than three days. If no relief is felt, change the remedy.

Conium Maculatum
Conditions from injuries and overexertion that sprain the left side of the sacroiliac symphysis. Cramp-like, aching and compressive pain in the

166

lower back, worse from bending backwards and twisting. It may feel as if there is a steel band around the sacrum. The pain prevents him turning in bed. It is worse from standing. The lower limbs may feel paralysed, and he staggers when he walks.

Dosage: One Conium 30c three times daily, for not more than three days. If no relief is felt, change the remedy.

Tellurium

This remedy is mainly for blows, falls and injuries that affect the sacrum. The right side of the sacroiliac symphysis is affected, and pains extend down the right thigh. Soreness is the main complaint. Touch hurts so much that he fears it, and avoids it. The back pain is worse on coughing or laughing.

Dosage: One Tellurium 30c three times daily, for not more than three days. If no relief is felt, change the remedy.

Variolinum

This is a good remedy for the effects of falls and injuries that are located in the sacrum. The pain is intolerable. It feels as if the back would break. The pain extends down the legs, and sometimes into the abdomen. Rising from a seat is so difficult and painful that he could faint. There is rheumatic pain in the muscles of the back. Movement is painful. He is very restless and tosses and turns at night in bed. Looks tired and complains of lack of sleep.

Dosage: One Variolinum 30c three times daily or as necessary for the pain, for not more than three days. Ruta and Rhus Tox. may also prove useful. If no relief is felt, change the remedy.

Coccyx Injuries

Hypericum

This is a very specific remedy for injuries to the coccyx, especially after a fall, and for fear following such injuries. The pain is violent and intolerable. Shooting and cutting, aching and soreness may all be present. The coccyx is painfully sensitive. There is spasm in the muscles. Sitting is extremely painful. There may also be some numbness following injury and concussion. Worse from movement.

Dosage: One Hypericum 30c daily for three days will help in most cases of injury to the spine. Arnica will also be needed after a fall.

Prolapsed Disc

The intervertebral disc is the weakest link of the lumbar spinal chain. Compression and torsion, as experienced in such widely different activities as driving in golf and scrummaging in rugby, weaken and may damage the annulus fibrosis, allowing extrusion of the nucleus. The onset may be sudden, following a match, or gradually over one or two days, following strenuous weight training or rowing. Sometimes the rigidity and pain arise during or following seemingly innocuous activity, such as bending over a table or bench, or lifting a light object, and is not confined to sports activity or dance.

Muscle spasm can be severe, and makes the person hold his back rigid. Any movement is fearfully painful. There may be more or less pain. It is commonly felt in the buttock and extends to the thigh. If the pain extends further down the leg, and there is sensory and/or motor dysfunction, neurological examination is essential and a surgical opinion may be needed urgently.

Rest on a firm mattress for two or three days may be necessary. When the spasm has decreased, gentle mobilising may accompany physiotherapy or osteopathy. Orthodox medicine recommends muscle relaxing drugs, anti-inflammatory drugs and possibly epidural injections of anaesthetic and steroids. Patients who do not wish to follow this route will find that correctly chosen homoeopathic remedies work swiftly and effectively to relieve the spasm, stiffness and pain.

CASE 29

John is a rugby prop forward. Two days after his last match of the season he was driving to work. He leaned forward to adjust the radio in the car, and described the feeling 'as if someone kicked me in the back'. He could not move, and was afraid to get out of his car. He drove to the clinic and struggled in to see me. It was rather amusing to hear him say, 'I'm OK really, but my back has given out.' I gave him one dose of Arnica 30c. He was immediately more relaxed and able to sit down. A colleague examined him and suspected a prolapsed disc, L3/4. He suggested that John did not require referral for X-rays at that time.

The pain was like sudden toothache, neuralgic, boring into his back, and radiated down the sciatic nerve. It made him cry out whenever he moved or was touched. He was afraid to move, and yet was restless. He said that he had been a bit chilled when he had a drink after the last match.

After a short time, and a second dose of Arnica, he felt well enough to be driven home where he went to bed.

He took some Magnesia Phosphorica 30c tablets with him to take as needed to relieve the muscle spasm. After a day's rest the spasm was very much reduced and he was more mobile. He felt that he could go back to work after two days.

John was left with some residual back pain. It was worse on first movement and at night. There was still some pain down the thigh at night. He found it difficult to find a comfortable position to sleep. Rhus Tox. 30c, one before bed for three nights, cured the problem. He kept a stock of this remedy to take as necessary. During the recovery he also received physiotherapy and followed a rehabilitation exercise routine.

Calcarea Carbonica

This tends to be the weightlifter's back remedy. The problem usually arises from overlifting. The back feels sprained and he cannot get up from a seat. He cannot sit up straight, and slumps in his seat. He has a sense of dislocation in the sacroiliac and looseness in the vertebrae, and his back is painful on pressure (compare to Sepia). He has shooting pains in the back that are worse at night, and when riding in a car or bus. It may hurt him to breathe. Any exertion makes him worse. Raw, cold air makes him worse, and immersion in cold water is very bad for him. He tends to be flabby, to wear loose clothes and to feel better if left to sit quietly.

Dosage: One Calc. Carb. 30c three times daily until he feels better, but for not more than three days. If no relief is felt, change the remedy.

Magnesia Phosphorica

This is the great homoeopathic antispasmodic remedy for cramps, convulsions and neuralgic pains. It is especially indicated when those conditions come on suddenly. The person is made worse by touch, getting cold and at night. It will relieve stiffness and cramps in the back. You may find that there is a pattern to the condition, and it may come on every two weeks, every six months or similarly. A typical picture is that the athlete or dancer reaches the end of a long, exhausting tournament, performance or season and, after relaxing, suddenly develops a prolapsed disc or spasm.

Dosage: If there are neuralgic spasms, one Mag. Phos. 30c three times a day, but for not more than three days. If no relief is felt, change the remedy.

Natrum Muriaticum

Almost the opposite of Rhus Tox., Natrum Mur. cannot straighten the back but can stoop easily. He has a feeling of paralysis in the lumbar region with painful stiffness. The spine is very sensitive. He has tearing pains that pulsate across his sacroiliac and into his hips. He complains of tension and pulling in his back. He has a bruised backache that is worse early in the morning and again between 10 and 11 a.m. It hurts to cough, and he is better when lying on his back on something hard. This person is worse from heat but enjoys massage. He does not like sympathy or fuss at all.

Dosage: One Natrum Mur. 30c three times daily, but for not more than three days. If no relief is felt, change the remedy.

Rhus Toxicodendron

Rhus Tox. is worse from first movement and better with continued movement. It is worse when sitting and lying. The back is stiff with painful tension when first moving. It is better from stretching, bending backwards and walking about, and also from lying on a hard surface. The pain extends into the thighs. Typically the person wakes early from the pain, cannot find a comfortable position in bed, is restless and cannot sleep. The pain extends down the sciatic nerve and makes him even more restless. He often has to get up early and walk around. Eventually he becomes exhausted mentally and physically, depressed and anxious.

Dosage: One Rhus Tox. 30c as necessary, but for not more than three days. If no relief is felt, change the remedy.

Sepia

The pain comes on suddenly, as if struck by a hammer. In the lumbar and sacral region the pain is burning, tearing and throbbing. Holds the lumbar spine rigid. It is very stiff. There is a dull ache in the lumbar spine, extending into the thighs. It is sore to touch, but hard pressure relieves it. Stands with the back pressed hard against something like a door jamb. It hurts to cough. It is worse when sitting. Walks about because it eases the pain. This person may have a history of back injury and weakness, because everything affects the back. Bending forward is painful. Worse from cold air. It is very strange, however, that this person, despite the injury, feels better during strenuous, even violent, exercise.

Dosage: One Sepia 30c as necessary for the pain, but for not more than three days. If no relief is felt, change the remedy.

The following case exemplifies how the right choice of remedy can hinge on a few symptoms. It is similar in circumstances to Case 29 above, but the remedy was different because the symptoms were peculiar to the case. Compare these two cases and the symptom pictures of Sepia and Mag. Phos.

CASE 30

David is my son. We were driving to the Alps for a climbing holiday when he was about thirty. We stopped for a coffee. He leaned forward in the car and shouted with pain. He said he felt as if someone had hit him in the sacrum with a large hammer, and his back felt rigid. I gave him Arnica 200c every fifteen minutes for five or six doses.

When we reached our overnight stop he was very stiff, had a dull ache in his back, and pain down his legs. Pressing his spine against something made it better. He had sat in the car with a hard cushion behind his back. He could not stoop or kneel, but wanted to go out for a good walk because he felt it would ease the pain and allow him to sleep. He was very anxious and felt that he had ruined our holiday. I gave him Sepia 30c, one tablet at 8 p.m. and another before bed. He slept well, and the following morning his back was much easier. He discontinued the remedy. It got much better over the next day, and we went on to climb a few mountains without any problems, or the need for any more Sepia.

Fractures in the Spine

Vertebral fractures due to traumatic sporting injury will usually respond to Arnica as a first remedy, and Symphytum will help fusion when the parts are back in position. The back remedies listed above may also help if the symptoms fit.

CASE 31

Mark is a rock climber who fell 30 feet during a climb. Falling backwards, he landed back first on hard rock. His dorsal spine was exceptionally painful and he was very shocked. Every movement, even being driven to hospital, was very painful. He was diagnosed as having fractured the spinus processes of T5 and T6. There being little that could be done, he was sent home and told to rest.

Mark had a rough night, relying on over-the-counter analgesics to deal with the pain. I was called the next day because he was in intolerable pain, and I prescribed Hypericum 30c, three doses. Later the same day he was feeling much better and could rest comfortably in bed. Every time he tried to move, however, the pain stopped him. It radiated from the centre of his back into both shoulders, and it made him afraid of moving. Going to the bathroom was problem. He wanted a bath because he felt it would make him feel better, but was afraid it would hurt too much.

I gave him Bryonia 30c to take, one every fifteen minutes. Within an hour he was able to get up and bathe without pain, and did feel better. I gave him more Hypericum 30c to take as needed to deal with the pain. With the pain under control he was able to go back to work in two days. He made a satisfactory recovery, and, five years later, is symptom-free.

Hypericum

This is a very specific remedy for injuries to the spine, as well as for fear following such injuries. The pain is violent and intolerable – shooting and cutting, aching and soreness between the scapulae. The spine is painfully sensitive. There is spasm in the muscles. There may also be some numbness following injury and concussion. He is worse from movement. It is one of the strange symptoms of Hypericum that the person often feels elated or 'on a high' before becoming injured.

Dosage: One or two doses of Hypericum 30c will help in most cases of injury to the spine. Arnica may also be needed after a fall.

THE CERVICAL SPINE

Fracture or Dislocation

Gymnastics, trampolining, diving, horseriding and rugby are sports that are particularly likely to lead to injuries to the cervical spine, because they involve activity that can end in falls with the head in flexion or extension. Legislation in contact sports is gradually eliminating such activities as spear tackling and dumping lock forwards in rugby, but the dangers of other actions and activities remain. There will always be a risk of rupture of stabilising ligaments and fracture of the vertebral arch, resulting in instability and a risk of cord damage and paralysis. Fortunately the injury is recognised in the majority of cases, and treated as serious with immobilisation and hospitalisation.

Sometimes an athlete or dancer walks in with a stiff neck and neurological symptoms, together with a story of trauma. Referral for medical opinion of the condition is essential. The possibility of fracture or dislocation should always be borne in mind, and X-ray, MRI and/or CT scans performed as appropriate to check for possible damage.

Arnica
This should be the first remedy for falls and similar trauma when the symptoms fit.
Dosage: One Arnica 30c hourly for three or four hours.

Hypericum
See opposite.

Symphytum
Dosage: See page 159.

Stiff Neck

It is possible that pain and stiffness in the neck could result from a prolapsed cervical disc. The pain ranges from a dull ache to very severe pain. Spasm may be very severe, blocking all cervical movement. Loss of sensation and reflex may be evident. If there are neurological signs, radiological examination should be done to eliminate bony lesions.

Although a collar may relieve pain and spasm, homoeopathic remedies can be used instead of muscle relaxants and NSAIDs to reduce the pain/spasm cycle and local tissue swelling. The remedies listed below will also serve to eliminate stiffness not due to trauma or overexertion.

The same remedies, chosen according to the symptoms, should be considered for whiplash injuries.

Anacardium
Stiffness with pain that is worse from motion. Dull pressure in neck and shoulders. Feels paralysed. After intense training or concentration.
Dosage: One Anacardium 30c to relieve the stiffness and pain. Repeat if necessary, but for not more than two days.

Calcarea Carbonica
Stiff neck after lifting, or after becoming cold when hot. Neck stiff and rigid. Hurts to breathe. Pressure hurts.
Dosage: One Calc. Carb. 30c to relieve the stiffness and pain. Repeat if necessary.

Rhododendron

Stiffness after getting wet or cold. Worse before storms, and early in the morning. Rheumatic and paralytic pains.

Dosage: One Rhododendron 30c to relieve the stiffness and pain. Repeat if necessary, but for not more than two days.

Rhus Toxicodendron

Usually the first remedy to use for a stiff neck. Wakes with it after strenuous exertion, getting cold when hot, or drafts. Stiff and painful on first moving but continued motion relieves. Very painful and tense. Better from hard pressure. Anxious and sad with the condition.

Dosage: One Rhus Tox. 30c to relieve the stiffness and pain. Repeat if necessary, but for not more than two days.

HEAD INJURIES

Trauma

It is an essential routine that anyone who is knocked unconscious should be taken to hospital for assessment and observation. This allows for prompt surgical intervention if there are signs of intracranial bleeding.

Even someone who has a suspected head injury but is not actually unconscious should be referred for medical investigation. Athletes can develop overuse head injuries as the result of repeated minor trauma and these must be thoroughly investigated.

Difficulties also arise when a player's loss of consciousness is so brief that it escapes notice, or if he or she remains conscious but suffers amnesia and confusion as the result of concussion. Repeated concussion can cause cumulative damage, leading to continuous confusion or 'punch-drunk' behaviour. Heading a football forcefully, punches in boxing, rugby scrummaging and similar activities can lead to repeated minor concussion.

All players suffering loss of consciousness or momentary confusion should stop the activity. If they complain of blurred vision, dizziness, nausea, vomiting and headache they should be questioned to elucidate whether there is confusion and retrograde amnesia. There is a danger that this condition may be associated with intracranial bleeding and cerebral contusion. There should be checks for variations in pupil size and limb mobility, and the player should be recommended for 24-hour observed bedrest. An observer should check regularly for changes in the mental or physical state.

There may be post-concussion symptoms of recurrent headaches, nausea, dizziness and difficult concentration, and these can last for six to eight weeks or even longer. Unless treated carefully such trauma can have a lifetime effect on the personality. Homoeopathic medicine can help to readjust the person's condition even a long time after the trauma.

Arnica
This remedy should be given in all cases of head injury or suspected head injury. Even the briefest loss of consciousness deserves a dose of Arnica. It will prevent intracranial bleeding and bruising, swelling and inflammation. The player will insist he is well and does not require treatment, but the astute physiotherapist or team manager will give him this remedy and insist that he leaves the field. If a player is unconscious from a head injury, give him Arnica by wetting his lips with a solution of the remedy in water. It may save serious repercussions and can promote recovery.
Dosage: One Arnica 30c as soon as possible.

Natrum Sulphuricum
This remedy will be useful when the symptoms following a head injury are longer lasting and persistent, possibly after medical opinion has been sought. There is dizziness with nausea and possibly vomiting. Confusion is marked, and the person develops a level of irritability that was not present before the injury. He becomes sensitive to noise and music, and suspicious. He may be depressed, even suicidal, but is too considerate of his family to commit suicide. Concentration on mental work makes him worse. His headache is crushing, bursting and nauseating. It may be throbbing and violent. He may also be very drowsy. His brain feels loose. He feels his head is in a vice. His headache is better if he lies down in a dark room. Most of his symptoms will be worse in the morning.

Give Natrum Sulph. in a potency according to the length of time following the injury: 30c a few days later; 200c, a few weeks later; 1M, months later; 10M a year or more later. Even years after a head injury, Natrum Sulph. in high potency will effectively cure many of the long-standing symptoms. This remedy is often prescribed for children who have suffered a long labour and birth process.
Dosage: One Natrum Sulph. 30c, 200c, 1M or 10M.

Opium

After complete loss of consciousness – and after medical opinion has been sought – when the person fears a repetition of the injury. He becomes very placid, apart from his fear, and says that there is nothing wrong with him (like Arnica). He is dreamy yet talkative, lacks will-power, or is nervous and irritable. He is light-headed after a head injury. His eyes may be glassy and staring, his pupils may be dilated or contracted or insensible to light. He falls into a heavy, coma-like sleep and snores loudly.

Dosage: One 200c potency of Opium to be taken every two hours for two days.

Scalp Injuries

Arnica

This remedy in tablet form will usually stop bleeding from a scalp wound. Do not apply topical Arnica to an open wound.

Dosage: One tablet of Arnica 30c every few minutes until the bleeding stops, and seek medical advice.

Calendula Cream

This cream helps to prevent infection and will promote healing.

Eye Injuries

Arnica

Dosage: One Arnica 30c tablet every three hours for a day following a blow to the eye will prevent discoloration, bruising and swelling.

Euphrasia

To relieve pain and soreness in an injured eye. This remedy will also relieve many eye symptoms such as discharge, soreness, conjunctivitis and pain, especially when there is profuse, hot and acrid watering.

Dosage: One Euphrasia 30c every few minutes for five doses.

Ledum

For bloodshot and bruised eyes. The top eyelid droops over the eye (ptosis).

Dosage: One Ledum 30c three times daily until the bruising begins to diminish, for a maximum of three days.

Symphytum
Follow Arnica with Symphytum 30c three times daily for three days to reduce swelling and discoloration.

Nose Injuries

Arnica
This is the first choice remedy for bleeding from a blow to the nose.
Dosage: One Arnica 30c tablet every three hours for a day following a blow to the nose will stop bleeding and prevent bruising and swelling.

Elaps Corallinus
If the nose continues to bleed dark-coloured blood after a blow. This remedy has the strange symptom that the nose bleeds in a room and stops when the person walks in the open air.
Dosage: One Elaps 30c for up to five doses.

Sepia
The nose bleeds from even a slight blow. The person may be very sensitive to smells, especially of food. Use this remedy if Arnica does not stop the bleeding after a few doses.
Dosage: One Sepia 30c every ten minutes for up to five doses.

Symphytum
This remedy will help the bones of a broken nose to heal once they have been set.
Dosage: One Symphytum 30c daily for two weeks.

Chapter 9

Treating Common Conditions

Sports people and dancers, indeed most physically active people, seem to be more susceptible to minor complaints than non-active people. Perhaps this is because they are more conscious of their bodies and general condition. The anxiety of performance naturally increases sensitivity to minor complaints, and tends to exaggerate them. It is generally accepted that moderate exercise enhances immune function, and there is some evidence that this is so, but Shephard and Shek (*Journal of Sports Medicine and Physical Fitness*, Vol. 34, No. 1, March 1994) report that exhausting exercise increases susceptibility to viral illnesses.

Overtraining in the weeks leading to competition, subclinical injuries in the working muscles, malnutrition and high levels of psychosocial stress all play their part in making athletes and dancers more prone to infections. *Fit to Dance?* suggests that dancers exercise for long periods without sufficient rest; that teachers and companies make excessive demands, both physical and psychological, on their dancers; that studio and theatre conditions, poor quality food and insufficient fluid intake all play their part in making dancers susceptible to viral infections. Many dancers demonstrate a depressed immune system that increases susceptibility to such illnesses as cold and flu. Fortunately, many dancers choose to turn first to complementary therapies for treatment when injured or sick.

Sportsmen and women who travel overseas to participate in their sports may be more susceptible to infections from unaccustomed food and drink.

Some of the most common complaints are listed below, together with suggestions for remedies from personal experience. If any of the following conditions persists it would be wise to consult a qualified and registered homoeopath or your doctor for professional help.

Alcohol

Most athletes are probably careful with alcohol but sometimes the post-match party can lead to misuse, overuse and hangovers. I wish I had known about Nux Vomica for hangovers in my rugby playing days!

If an athlete or dancer is addicted to alcohol or drugs, a homoeopath could help with the treatment on a constitutional level.

Nux Vomica

To avoid hangovers, take one tablet of Nux Vomica 30c before going to bed and one first thing in the morning. Drink a glass of water at about the same time. I have known one Nux Vomica 30c, given to someone who had drunk far too much beer, act as an emetic. Unfortunately it worked within ten seconds, well before the person could get to the bathroom. The following morning he was well enough to go to work.
Dosage: One Nux Vom. 30c and a glass of water before bed. Repeat in the morning if the hangover persists.

Altitude

The early effects of altitude on sports performance seem worse for endurance events than for power events. The immediate effects are shortage of breath and increased frequency of breathing, increased pulse rate, loss of appetite and insomnia. Lassitude and increased tiredness are common. Most people become acclimatised within two days or so. Mountaineers and skiers probably suffer the worst effects, which include nausea, sore throat, joint pains and severe headaches. A short hacking cough can be an early sign of acute mountain sickness, which is a serious condition. Take the person down at least 600m as soon as possible. Coca is an excellent homoeopathic remedy for the effects of altitude which I have used successfully many times.

Altitude can affect the breathing, endurance and performance of players, athletes and dancers at levels of 5,500 ft (1,500 m) and higher if they are unaccustomed to performing at those altitudes. Coca will both resolve the problems associated with altitude and boost energy and endurance:

Coca

Shortage of breath, breathing becomes fast and difficult, especially in older athletes. Short hacking cough generated by tickling and irritation in the larynx. This cough becomes paroxysmal and debilitating, and

179

the person can faint from the weakness. If the cough is productive there will be yellow phlegm. Headache in the forehead and occiput, or either, that is aggravated by coughing. There may be vertigo, violent palpitations, nosebleeds, nausea and hoarseness. Sleep is disturbed and restless, with many dreams. One of the strange effects of altitude is that people can become elated and euphoric, and these are mental symptoms of this remedy. It is also valuable against the effects of a long flight. Exhaustion and prostration are also symptoms.

Dosage: One Coca 30c as soon as the symptoms appear.

Anxiety

See pages 288–90 for a full treatment of pre-performance anxiety.

Arsenicum Album

For the person who is generally anxious, much worse at night and in bed, is restless, and moves from place to place, is oversensitive, fault-finding and fastidious, and anxious on waking.

Dosage: One Arsenicum 30c taken before bed will help him to calm down and have a good night.

Asthma

It is essential that anyone suffering from asthma, or suspected asthma, should be under medical care. Homoeopathic constitutional prescribing is often very successful with asthma.

There has been a surprising increase in asthma among sports people in recent years. Homoeopaths have been treating asthma successfully for over a hundred years, and the sufferer should be advised to consult a professional homoeopath. It is likely that they are already using inhalers such as Ventolin. They should not be advised to stop using them. There is some suggestion that Ventolin, by decreasing airways resistance, may enhance performance. If an athlete has an asthma attack he may need to be hospitalised urgently. Do not hesitate or meddle with homoeopathic or any other remedies before referring him.

There are a few acute remedies with a known affinity to this illness.

Antimonium Tartaricum

This is an excellent remedy for strengthening the lungs and clearing mucus when there is weakness and drowsiness and the person is too weak to bring up the phlegm, which is thick and white. The chest

180

rattles. Asthma sometimes brought on by too much tea, coffee or alcohol. Irritable.

Dosage: One Ant. Tart. 6c three times daily for not more than seven days.

Arsenicum Album

Asthma since childhood, possibly with a long history of bronchitis and respiratory infections. This remedy will be useful for the person who wakes between 1 a.m. and 2 a.m. with shortness of breath and having to sit up to breathe. Great anxiety, restlessness, cold sweat, whistling and wheezing. Much worse from cold, but needs fresh air. Fears suffocation. This person is quick, alive, restless and fussy.

Dosage: One Arsenicum 30c before bed for three nights and as necessary during an attack.

Ipecacuanha

Constriction of chest and larynx, gasping for breath, incessant paroxysms of violent cough with nausea. Loose rattle in chest without phlegm. Worse damp and motion. Immediately better in the open air, and from resting.

Dosage: One Ipecac. 30c before bed for three nights.

Athlete's Foot

Calendula Cream

Will reduce the inflammation effectively.

Graphites

When the folds between the toes become raw and moist and exude a gluey, honey-like moisture.

Dosage: One Graphites 6c, three times daily by mouth for not more than three days, or until the condition begins to improve. One pill may be dissolved in water to make a lotion to bathe the feet and wash between the toes.

Hypercal Cream

Will prevent itching and reduce the inflammation.

Psorinum

If the symptoms are similar to Sulphur but the person is cold.

Dosage: As for Sulphur.

Rescue Remedy Cream
This Bach remedy will also help to relieve the itching and inflammation.

Silica
Cracks between the toes, slow inflammation, suppurative, itching and painful, with much smelly sweat.
Dosage: One Silica 30c tablet daily for a few days until the condition begins to improve. Dissolve one tablet in enough water to bathe the feet in twice a day.

Warning: Do not give Silica above the 6c potency if the patient has synthetic tissue of any sort in his body. A replacement hip, a polytetrafluoroethylene (PTFE) repair to a cruciate ligament, or even a pacemaker may be rejected following Silica in high potency.

Sulphur
If there is more itching at night in bed, and the feet are burning hot. The skin may burn when scratched and there may be excoriation between the toes. Use the lotion to bathe the feet and between the toes. The person who needs Sulphur may not have as clean feet as you would wish, and will be hot and sweaty.
Dosage: Sulphur 6c, one daily by mouth for three days, or dissolved in water to make a lotion to bathe the feet.

Black Eye

Arnica
Dosage: One Arnica 30c after a blow to the eye, to prevent a black eye developing.

Ledum Palustre
When the eyes are bruised and bloodshot, ache, and are worse at night when warm.
Dosage: One Ledum 30c three times daily until the bruising begins to disappear, for not more than three days.

Symphytum
Injuries to the eye from blunt instruments or blows. The eye closes spasmodically and there are shooting pains.

182

Dosage: One Symphytum 30c three times daily until the bruising begins to disappear, for not more than three days.

Bleeding

Arnica

Arnica by mouth will often stop minor bleeding quickly.
Dosage: Whatever potency available as frequently as necessary to stop the bleeding. Probably two doses, up to a maximum of six doses.

Phosphorus

When the bleeding is profuse and the blood is bright red and restarts easily, and Arnica does not help.
Dosage: Phosphorus 30c every few minutes until it stops, for five doses maximum.

Blisters

The best treatment for blisters is the earliest one. As soon as a hot spot develops it should be treated with Bach Rescue Remedy cream and protected with tape. If the blister has already developed, puncture it with a sterilised needle and drain the ampoule, leaving the skin as intact as possible. Apply Bach Rescue Remedy cream and protect with over-lapping layers of zinc oxide tape. Leave the tape in place for as long as the exercise continues. Apply Calendula cream to prevent infection when the tape is removed.

There are two remedies and one cream that may help relieve the pain of blisters.

Cantharis

Smarting, burning, raw pain with violent inflammation. Strangely the pain is better from rubbing and warmth. The blisters themselves burn when touched, and may be better from applying cold water.
Dosage: Cantharis 30c, one tablet hourly for pain for six doses, and one dissolved in water to make a lotion to bathe the sore parts.

Urtica Urens

Stinging, burning pain, worse from cold bathing and touch.
Dosage: Urtica 30c, one tablet hourly for pain for six doses, and one dissolved in water to make a lotion to bathe the sore parts.

Calendula Cream
Apply topically to prevent infection and to promote rapid healing.

Burns (see also **Sunburn**)

Causticum
Deep burns that itch painfully and are very sore and raw. The shock
from burns responds to this remedy. Colds and drafts make the pain
worse.
Dosage: One Causticum 30c tablet every two hours for a maximum of
seven doses.

Urtica Urens
The ointment is an excellent remedy for minor burns.
Dosage: One Urtica 30c tablet every few hours in one day will ease the
stinging pain from burns.

Cold Sores

Someone who has frequent cold sores may need a constitutional
remedy. A good emergency treatment for cold sores is to bathe them
with instant coffee dissolved in cold water.

Calendula
Use the cream for sore lips.

Graphites
When the lips are cracked and sore from cold.
Dosage: One Graphites 30c. Dissolve one in water and bathe the lips
with it.

Natrum Muriaticum
For persistent cracks in the middle of the lower lip. For cold sores on
the lips and around the mouth from tiredness, stress, anxiety and exposure to sun.
Dosage: One Natrum Mur. 30c, twice daily for three days.

Rhus Toxicodendron
Crusty, itching and burning cold sores around the mouth. They are
worse in the morning on waking.
Dosage: Rhus Tox. 30c, three times daily for three days.
For persistent painful cracks in the middle of the lower lip.

Urtica Urens
Burned, sore, smarting lips from exposure to the sun. Use the ointment.

Common Cold

A combination of Aconite 6c, Belladonna 6c and Chamomilla 6c, taken at the first signs of a cold, will relieve the symptoms and may keep the cold to a minimum. It is especially relevant if the cold follows a chill.
Dosage: One tablet of each remedy as soon as the cold appears. There is usually no need to repeat.

Allium Cepa
The cold comes on after exposure to biting cold damp wind. There is a constant drip of copious watery discharge and the nose is red and raw. Generally hot and thirsty, and worse in the evening and indoors.
Dosage: One Allium Cepa 6c tablet three times daily for three days.

Arsenicum Album
For the person who has many colds, notices drafts, and suffers most in cold damp weather. The cold starts in the nose and quickly goes to the throat and chest, producing a hard, dry tickling cough. Thirsty, restless, weak and needs warmth.
Dosage: One Arsenicum 6c tablet three times in one day.

Gelsemium
For a cold that takes several days to develop, and is slow to come on. Or for a cold with the symptoms of flu that comes on suddenly. Sneezing, red face, heavy eyelids, cold limbs, aching in all joints, headache and drowsiness. Gelsemium is probably the most used remedy for flu.
Dosage: One Gelsemium 6c to prevent flu. If you have flu, one 30c three times in one day.

Hepar Sulphuris
Sneezing from uncovering, even putting an arm out of bed makes him sneeze. Very sensitive to draughts and cold wind. Nasal catarrh drips down the back of the throat and is yellow and smelly. The bones of the nose feel sore and the sense of smell may be lost.
Dosage: One Hepar Sulph. 6c tablet three times in one day.

Natrum Muriaticum

The nose runs 'like a tap', gushing hot watery discharge, and early morning sneezing.

Dosage: One Natrum Mur. 6c as soon as the symptoms appear.

Nux Vomica

Sneezing, runny nose during the day that blocks up at night, better in the open air, worse in the morning. He is irritable, has a headache, sore throat and a very runny nose.

Dosage: One Nux Vom. 6c three times daily for three days.

Confidence (Lack of)

Homoeopaths tend to use the higher potencies for emotional and mental symptoms. See also Chapter 12.

Baryta Carbonica

Shy, timid, especially among strangers, thinks he is being laughed at and made fun of, avoids company and does not want to socialise. Loses self-confidence. He can be very childish in behaviour, and this some-times gets him into trouble. Not to be confused with nervousness and anxiety before an event, this person is fundamentally and childishly shy and nervous.

Dosage: One Baryta Carb. 200c three times daily for three days.

Lycopodium

Loses self-confidence when faced with doing something new, or per-forming in a new environment. For example, playing on a ground that is new to him. Becomes angry, anxious and hurried. Very nervous before playing or performing, but always does well and overcomes the nerves as the game begins. Enjoys the challenge of new places, but sometimes the anxiety and self-doubt become too much and affect per-formance adversely.

Dosage: Lycopodium 200c, two or three doses before or during the match to settle nerves and restore confidence.

Silica

Loss of self-confidence in anticipation of an event. Unlike Lycopodium and Baryta Carb., this person is afraid of failure and its consequences. He is also very obstinate. He will decide he is not going to play, and nothing will shake that resolve. Yet, in other ways, and when confident, he is most cooperative and agreeable. This conflict between confidence and insecurity is typical of the person who would benefit from Silica.

Dosage: One dose of Silica 10M. Watch the confidence grow as the conflict diminishes.

Warning: As stated already in this book, do not give Silica above the 6c potency if the patient has synthetic tissue of any sort in his body. A replacement hip, a polytetrafluoroethylene (PTFE) repair to a cruciate ligament, or even a pacemaker may be rejected following Silica in high potency.

Constipation

Chronic or regular constipation should always be referred to the general practitioner in the first instance. You may then wish to seek treatment from a qualified homoeopath. He or she will prescribe the constitutional remedy to alleviate the problem. There are a few specific remedies which may help temporary constipation.

Lac Defloratum

Constipation with ineffectual urging and great straining to pass a large hard stool. Pain radiates from below the sternum and across the abdomen at about the level of the umbilicus. Violent sick headache. There is much stinking flatus that relieves his pain. Milk aggravates the condition and produces nausea.

Dosage: One Lac Defloratum 30c three times daily for up to a week.

Nux Vomica

Uneasy feeling in the bowels with ineffectual urging to defecate. The bowels seem inactive, and would feel better if only he could go. Tenderness and cutting pain in the lower abdomen. Irritable, sometimes irrationally so, when constipated, and really does feel better after a successful stool. The constipation is usually associated with eating strange food and drinks on foreign tours, and other stomach upsets, indigestion, heartburn and aversion to food.

Dosage: Nux Vomica 30c, one tablet every morning until the system settles down to routine, for not more than seven days.

Opium

This is an effective remedy for constipation when there is absolutely no desire for stool and no urging. Constipation from hot weather. There is throbbing in the abdomen and a feeling as if the anus were closed. The bowels feel completely obstructed and paralysed. Cannot even pass flatus although the abdomen feels distended and hard, and as if there was a weight inside. Placid, dull, sluggish and lacks willpower when constipated, and talkative, happy and lively when he is well.

Dosage: Opium 30c three times daily for two days may help, but beware – Opium can produce temporary incontinence of faeces.

Coughs

There are many homoeopathic remedies that treat coughs effectively. There are a few that may be effective for acute coughs in physically active people. To choose the remedy, listen to the cough, look at the person, ask about the pain – what makes it worse, and at what time of day, and where there is a tickle, if any.

Some of the remedies I have used successfully for acute coughs are listed below.

Dosage: Use the indicated remedies in the 6c potency. Dissolve one tablet under the tongue every few minutes until relief is felt. If the remedy does not ease the cough after five or six doses, try the next indicated one.

For chronic, long-lasting coughs it is important to be under medical supervision as well as to consult a qualified homoeopath.

Aconite

For a short dry painful barking cough brought on suddenly by exposure to dry cold conditions or being chilled. It is worse in the evening or at night, and aggravated by breathing, smoking and drinking. It should be the first remedy to try after becoming chilled. Grasps the throat when coughing. Very anxious and restless.

Bryonia

Coughing from the slightest movement, even breathing. All he wants to do is to lie still and immobile. He holds his chest when he coughs because he feels it will explode. Dry, very painful cough, worse at night and generated by tickling in the larynx. Wants to be left alone and does not want to talk.

Drosera

Rapid, deep, barking, violent, prolonged and incessant cough that is worse after midnight and prevents sleep. Coughing every time he lies down. Deep hoarse voice. Difficult to speak. Also holds the chest when coughing, but can move around. Because it is worse when he lies down he tends to walk about. This helps to differentiate Drosera from Bryonia. This cough follows a cold and sore throat. As if a feather is tickling the throat. Drosera will often clear up a persistent cough following a common cold.

Hepar Sulphuris

A barking cough that produces much mucus, but it is difficult to bring up. There is much rattling in the chest, and then he gets up thick yellow phlegm. Hates draughts and cold air, which makes the cough worse. Very irritable. Look out for the person who tells you irritably to close a door or window.

Phosphorus

A dry hard cough with tickling behind the sternum. It wakes the person at night, and he has to sit up to cough. Going from a warm room out into the cold air aggravates the cough. Cold drinks ease it, but are vomited a short time later. Prostrated and exhausted by the cough. Pain in the abdomen, with wheezing, burning in the air passages and trembling. Loves sympathy.

Rumex

Extremely sensitive to cold air. Keeps a blanket or towel over the head and face to prevent him from breathing the cold air. Every breath of cold air causes tickling in the throat pit and a continuous cough. Wakes in the morning with a dry, hacking cough. Worse in cold air, and from going from a warm room to a cold one, or vice versa. Breathing, lying down, night-time, talking and uncovering all make the cough worse. There is pain under the sternum. Very restless. He may cover his mouth with his hands, even when he is not coughing. This would be my first choice for a dry, hacking cough.

Spongia

The Spongia cough is very distinctive. It is croupy and sounds like someone sawing thin board. It is very rough, hollow and barking. Feels as if there is a sponge, leaves or tissue in the larynx, and the breath has

189

to go through it. Excitement can bring on this cough. Warm drinks and food relieve it briefly, as does sitting up. The voice is hoarse and the larynx painful dry and constricted. Breathing is deep, and may sound loud between bouts of coughing, and the person may fear that he has asthma or some other serious illness.

Cramps

Muscle cramp is a common, painful, physiological disturbance of skeletal muscle suffered by many athletes and dancers. It is a severe, sudden, involuntary and sustained contraction of the muscle and can be extremely painful. Exercise-induced muscle cramp is unpredictable and is a frustrating problem for that reason. It affects a wide range of performers and athletes, ranging from the unfit person who undertakes sudden unaccustomed exertion to the highly trained and conditioned athlete or dancer who incurs extended and prolonged vigorous activity in circumstances of increased stress, such as a cup final or an exceptionally demanding performance.

Orthodox treatment for cramp is by reflex inhibition and afferent stimulation. For example, calf cramp is resolved by stretching the leg with the foot dorsiflexed. Muscle stretching, correction of muscle balance, adequate conditioning, mental preparation and avoidance of provocative drugs may be beneficial. Several homoeopathic remedies that have been used successfully to treat and prevent cramps are listed below.

Older people may suffer cramps in bed at night. These cases should be referred to a doctor or professional homoeopath for help.

There is a very good acupressure treatment for cramp in the calf. Find the hollow between the two big calf muscles, about half way between the bend in the knee and the top of the heel, and press hard in that spot with your thumb for a few seconds.

Calcarea Carbonica
Cramps in the calves when stretching out the legs at night after physical exertion during the day. Legs and feet are cold and clammy. Tired from least exertion.
Dosage: One Calc. Carb. 30c before bed for up to seven nights.

Cuprum
Violent cramps in the calves after strenuous physical activity and exertion. The muscles are knotted. Stretching them relieves the intense pain.

Dosage: One dose of Cuprum 30c before a very demanding event will prevent their onset. Taken when cramps begin, it will prevent recurrence.

Magnesia Phosphorica
Cramps from prolonged exertion, especially in the calf. Rubbing relieves them. Always talking about injuries and pains.
Dosage: One Mag. Phos. 30c if prolonged exertion is expected. One dose dissolved in warm water may be drunk each evening for a few days if someone has regular cramps at night.

In order to prevent cramp take one Mag. Phos. 30c and one Cuprum 30c before an arduous and potentially prolonged event.

Diarrhoea (Food Poisoning)

Prevention
Teams playing overseas sometimes suffer 'tummy troubles', which usually means, nausea, sickness and diarrhoea. If one takes sensible precautions they need not interfere with an overseas tour. These are:

1) Do not drink or clean teeth in suspect water. In Africa and Asia all water is suspect. Use only boiled, purified or bottled mineral water.
2) Do not eat salads or other cold food that has been washed in tap water.
3) Do not eat ice cream, food, cakes or puddings that are not fresh.
4) Wash all fruit in boiled, purified or bottled water, and peel it.
5) Check that all food has been thoroughly cooked. Ask them to reheat it if necessary.
6) Do not take ice in drinks.

Treatment
Even the best precautions cannot prevent some diarrhoea. If you have diarrhoea the best course of action to take is:

1) Stop eating for at least 24 hours.
2) Drink as much boiled, purified or bottled mineral water as possible.
3) Take one or more of the homoeopathic remedies listed below.
4) A good test of when you can start eating again is when you can break wind safely.

Dosage: One of the following remedies in the 6c or 30c potency, one tablet every hour for up to five or six doses. If the remedy does not stop the diarrhoea, try the next indicated remedy.

Arsenicum Album

This is the first remedy to choose if the diarrhoea is from contaminated food. There are violent cramping pains across the abdomen, and the stools are burning, watery, offensive, frequent and possibly involuntary. They may contain undigested food. The stool burns the anus as it passes. The person is cold, shivery and restless. Wants to sip frequent cold drinks. Very anxious, says 'I wish I was dead.' Very restless and cannot stay in his bed. Wanders around. Sudden weakness.

China

Painless diarrhoea, usually during hot weather. The stools are dark, watery, foul, and consist mainly of undigested food. The diarrhoea is preceded by flatulent bloating and colic. You may suspect it was caused by fruit, milk or beer, especially in hot weather. There may be drenching cold sweats when the person is at stool, and terrible weakness.

Colocynthis

Violent, cutting, gripping, clutching, colicky pains that come in waves across abdomen. Watery, yellow, shreddy, painful stools squirt out. Following the least food or drink, and renewed whenever he eats. The pains make him bend double to relieve them.

Podophyllum

Diarrhoea preceded by a terrible gurgling through the bowels. Then profuse putrid stool gushes out painlessly and without warning. Worse in hot weather. This is worst in the early morning.

Notes

1) It may be necessary to prescribe remedies rapidly one after another as the symptoms change.
2) If diarrhoea continues, consult your doctor. A homoeopath may then be able to help to alleviate the problem.

Diarrhoea (Nervous)

Argentum Nitricum

For nervous diarrhoea before a match or performance. The person has to evacuate the bowels urgently and sometimes frequently. Urinating also becomes more frequent and urgent. He is nervous, anxious, impulsive and hurried.

Dosage: One Arg. Nit. 30c the night before, and repeated one hour before the event, can alleviate the problem.

Epistaxis (Nosebleed)

Arnica
Bleeding from a blow to the nose. Chronic nosebleeds persisting some time following a blow to the nose. Coughing, sneezing and blowing the nose all make it bleed. After exertion. After washing the face. At altitude.
Dosage: One Arnica 30c taken as necessary to stop the bleeding, for three doses.

Elaps Corallinus
If the nose continues to bleed dark coloured blood after a blow. This remedy has the strange symptom that the nose bleeds in a room and stops when the person walks in the open air.
Dosage: One Elaps 30c daily for three doses.

Hamamelis
Morning nosebleeds of thin dark blood. Tranquil person.
Dosage: One Hamamelis 30c daily for three doses.

Phosphorus
Chronic and persistent epistaxis of bright red blood, perhaps with clots. Brought on by blowing the nose, exertion, sweating, rubbing the nose. Especially for young people who seem to have grown too fast.
Dosage: One Phosphorus 30c three times daily for three days.

Sepia
The nose bleeds from even a slight blow. The person may be very sensitive to smells, especially of food. Use this remedy if Arnica does not stop the bleeding after a few doses.
Dosage: One Sepia 30c every ten minutes for up to three doses.

Exhaustion

See Chapter 12 for remedies to improve endurance.

Arnica

I have found that one Arnica 30c taken as soon as you begin to feel tired will prevent exhaustion.

Coca

This remedy has the reputation for giving a boost to a tired athlete or dancer.

Dosage: One Coca 30c.

Picric Acid

For the person who is totally exhausted in body and mind, and is weak, tired and feels heavy. Wants only to rest. Lacks the will power to attempt anything yet deeply fears failure. Aching, tired limbs. Sleepless from exhaustion; sleeps only restlessly, and feels 'too tired to sleep'.

Dosage: One Picric Acid 200c.

Flying

Borax

For fear of flying. The person is badly affected by the upward and downward motion of flying, is nervous, anxious, irritable, fidgety, and starts or is frightened by sudden noise. He has vertigo, his ears feel closed up and he has wind. Sleeps badly and wakes at 4 a.m. Pain in ears and sinuses after flying.

Dosage: One Borax 30c the day before flying, and another one hour before and every hour during the flight.

Coca

This remedy counteracts the effects of long periods at an altitude of between 5,000 ft and 8,000 ft – the cabin pressurisation of most airlines.

Dosage: One Coca 30c the day before flying, one an hour before and every hour during the flight.

Food Poisoning (see Diarrhoea, pages 191–2)

Gout

Antimonium Crudum
Extreme tenderness of feet. Very irritable and fretful, and tends to have an upset stomach too.
Dosage: One Ant. Crud. 200c tablet daily for three days.

Arnica
Fears being touched, bruised pain in toe from blow. Injury to toe becomes gouty.
Dosage: Arnica 200c, one tablet daily for three days.

Colchicum Autumnale
This is the main remedy for gout. Cannot bear touch to foot. The part swells oedematously. Worse for the slightest movement, cold, and at night. Tearing pain in toe and foot, with swelling. Depressed, irritable and sensitive to pain and disturbance.
Dosage: One Colchicum 30c or 200c tablet daily for three days.

Urtica Urens
Burning pain, worse in cool damp weather.
Dosage: One Urtica 30c or 200c tablet daily for three days.

Grass Burns

Calendula Cream
Prevents infection and promotes healing.

Urtica Urens Ointment
Intense burning pain. Prevents blistering.

Haemorrhoids (see **Piles,** page 206–7)

Hangover (see **Alcohol,** page 179)

Hay Fever

If the following remedies do not relieve the condition after five or six doses, a qualified homoeopath will be able to prescribe more effectively for the condition.

Allium Cepa

The eyes stream with water, but they are not sore. The nose streams with water, and becomes very sore. There is frequent violent sneezing and a raw sore throat. It is worse in the spring and in August, and in a warm room.

Dosage: One Allium Cepa 30c every day during the worst time of year, and every two hours when the symptoms are at their most troublesome.

Euphrasia

This remedy is best for hay fever when the nasal discharge is profuse but bland, and the hot watery discharge from the eyes makes them – and even the cheeks – very sore and red (the opposite of Allium Cepa). It is worse in sunshine and wind.

Dosage: One Euphrasia 30c every day during the worst time of year, and every two hours when the symptoms are at their most troublesome.

Sabadilla

The symptoms come on regularly at set periods, every two or four weeks, or at the same time every year. There is persistent violent sneezing with itching and tickling in the nose. The nose runs with watery discharge. It is worse from the smell of flowers, and even from the thought of flowers. The eyelids are red and burning and watering. It is better in the open air and the person tends to be miserable with the condition.

Dosage: One Sabadilla 30c every day during the worst time of year, and every two hours when the symptoms are at their worst.

Headache

There are 272 remedies that could cure a headache! Here are a few that could help.

Dosage: One tablet of the indicated remedy in 6c or 30c potency should be taken every hour for a maximum of six doses. Stop when the headache ceases or begins to recede.

Belladonna, Glonoine

Headache from too much sun.

Bryonia
Headache comes on during the night and he wakes with it, worse from any movement, holds his head with the pain.

Coca
Headache after a long flight.

Cocculus
Headache with nausea, especially when travelling by boat or car.

Lachesis
Headache comes on as he opens his eyes in the morning, mainly left sided, from exposure to heat and sun, talks a lot.

Natrum Muriaticum
Headache from excitement, comes on between 9 and 11 a.m.

Natrum Sulphuricum
Headache after a head injury, even a very long time after.

Nux Vomica
Headache after breakfast, at 3 a.m., after drinking too much alcohol or eating too much rich food.

Pulsatilla
Headache, pulsating, one-sided, from stuffy warm room, worse from lying down, better for gentle walking in the open air.

Sulphur
Headache with nausea, comes on regularly every seven days, worse from standing and bathing.

Heat (Weather Conditions)

Exertion in unaccustomed hot conditions can result in cramp, exhaustion or heatstroke. For the homoeopathic treatment of cramp refer to the section above. The following remedies will treat heat exhaustion effectively.

Antimonium Crudum
This remedy will help athletes, dancers and performers who have to cope with unaccustomed hot weather and are badly affected by it.

Better in the open air and when lying down to rest. Loses appetite, may be nauseous and has a disordered stomach. Fretful, cross and peevish, or dreamy and sentimental. Upset by dirt and mess. Very sleepy and weary in hot weather. Avoids any exertion.

Dosage: One Ant. Crud. 30c tablet as soon as symptoms become evident. Repeat the remedy hourly until feeling better, or for six doses maximum.

Kali Bichromicum

Use this remedy if the person responds to hot weather by feeling indifferent and averse to mental and physical work, and avoids other people. Sleep is difficult and he may wake at 2 to 3 a.m. and be unable to sleep again. Strangely this person may normally be chilly in himself, and dislike the cold, even when he complains of the heat! Better from moving around, may suffer flushes of heat and the sweat will be sticky.

Dosage: One Kali Bich. 30c hourly for six doses.

Heatstroke

Heatstroke is a serious condition requiring medical attention. The skin becomes dry and hot, sweating ceases, the body temperature rises to dangerous levels and death can result. It is particularly dangerous in long distance endurance events such as marathon running. There are two homoeopathic remedies that can be used to treat the athlete.

Belladonna

The person needing Belladonna is burning hot, so hot that you feel your fingers burning after touching him. He is bright red and very dry, will have a great thirst for cold water and may have an awful throbbing, hammering headache. Any exposure to the sun makes him feel worse, and he cannot stand being touched. Any jarring motion will make him complain. I have known a Belladonna patient complain from the jarring as I walked across the bedroom floor. He may be very delirious and restless, and may become unusually quarrelsome. He cannot sleep, and when he does he dreams horrible dreams of murder, fire and quarrels.

Dosage: One Belladonna 6c or 30c.

Glonoine

This remedy is the first choice in every case of heat stroke and heat exhaustion. He complains of violent pulsation, and cannot bear heat especially on his head. He will do anything to avoid the heat of the sun, and is desperate to rest in the shade. Any movement makes him worse. He has waves of terrible, pounding, bursting headache, and feels as if his blood is all in his head. He is confused and bewildered. If he continues activity in the heat of the sun he may fall unconscious. There will be a blueness about his face, and he may clench his jaws tightly. He has flushes of heat, with hot sweat.

Dosage: Glonoine 6c three doses repeated as necessary. I recommend using it prophylactically, taking it one day before an event in exceptionally hot sunny weather, one hour before the start and in solution in any drinks taken during the event. If the patient is unconscious, wet his lips and bathe his wrists with a solution of Glonoine 30c or 200c.

Homesickness

Not only children suffer from homesickness. It can affect an athlete's or dancer's performance during quite short trips abroad or while away from home.

Capsicum

Homesickness with sleeplessness, changeable moods, laughing and weeping in turn, sentimental, nostalgic, peevish and irritable, wants to be left alone. Dislikes draughts and feels better with continued movement. Feels much worse at bedtime.

Dosage: One Capsicum 200c.

Phosphoric Acid

This is the most specific remedy for homesickness. The person becomes quiet, apathetic and brooding. Becomes emotional, disinterested and tired. May be sleepy during the day but sleeps badly at night.

Dosage: One Phosphoric Acid 200c.

Indigestion

Lycopodium

Feels very hungry, but is full after a few mouthfuls. Becomes very bloated with wind. Burning, acid pain in stomach with burning wind. Bread, soup, pasta and cold foods disagree with him. He prefers warm food. He suffers from nervous indigestion before a match or performance and eats only little.

Dosage: One Lycopodium 30c.

199

Nux Vomica
The food lies like a stone in the stomach. Indigestion after eating rich food and drinking alcohol, coffee and late nights. Acid risings into the throat. Better after a hot drink, and from vomiting. Very irritable, angry and impatient. Many foods disagree. Usually the first choice for indigestion.
Dosage: One Nux Vomica 30c.

Pulsatilla
Indigestion from fats, rich foods, toast, onions, tobacco smoke, tea, ice cream, cakes, warm food and drink. Comes on long after eating. Better in the open air. Differentiate from Nux Vomica by the personality. The Pulsatilla person is mild-mannered, easy-going and enjoys sympathy, but can be very emotional and change moods easily.
Dosage: One Pulsatilla 30c.

Influenza

See symptoms and remedies in the 'Common Cold' section (pages 185–6).

Ingrowing Toenail

Calendula Cream
Will eradicate the infection associated with this condition without the need for antibiotics. A more roomy toe box in shoes will remove the causation. Refer to a chiropodist for chronic ingrowing toenails.

Graphites
Thick, rough ingrowing nails. Cold, wet feet. Toes chafed by sweat.
Dosage: One Graphites 6c, three times daily by mouth for one week.

Silica
Yellow, distorted nails. Offensive foot sweat. Icy cold and sweaty. Toes and soles sore.
Dosage: One Silica 6c, three times daily by mouth for one week.

Insomnia

China
From fantasies – 'building castles in the air'. Thoughts crowd the mind. Irritable, very touchy, avoids company. Insomnia returns at set periods.

Dosage: One China 30c before bed. Repeat if sleep does not come, for up to three doses.

Coffea Cruda

From excitement, nervous energy, mental activity, hearing every sound, becomes irritable from wakefulness.
Dosage: One Coffea 30c tablet in the early evening, and one before bed.

Noctura

Nelson's Homoeopathic Pharmacy produces this very good combination remedy for insomnia. Available from most large pharmacies.
Dosage: Follow the directions on the packaging.

Nux Vomica

Cannot sleep from rush of ideas, or wakes very early, about 3 a.m., and cannot get to sleep again.
Dosage: One Nux Vomica 30c tablet before bed. Repeat if waking at around 3 a.m.

Picric Acid

Too exhausted and tired to be able to sleep.
Dosage: One Picric Acid 200c before bed.

Pulsatilla

Thoughts go round and round in the head. Frequent waking, restless, anxious dreams. Overactive mind.
Dosage: One Pulsatilla 30c tablet before bed.

Rescue Remedy

I have often prescribed a few drops of this Bach flower remedy for insomnia with good effect.
Dosage: Place a few drops beneath the tongue before bed.

Mouth Ulcers

Borax
For painful, sensitive ulcers on the tongue that bleed easily.
Dosage: One Borax 30c three times daily for three days.

Mercurius Solubilis
Painful ulcers in the cheeks and gums and behind the lips, with much salivation and really offensive bad breath. The teeth make indentations in the tongue.
Dosage: One Mercurius 30c every hour for three doses.

Nitric Acid
Ulcers with sharp, splinter-like pains, putrid breath and salivation. Ulcers in soft palate and gums. Green coating on tongue.
Dosage: One Nitric Acid 30c every hour for three doses.

Nausea (see also **Diarrhoea,** pages 191–3)

There are many remedies for nausea. I suggest here a few that are particularly appropriate for sports persons.
Dosage: The remedy should be chosen and taken once or twice in the 30c potency to relieve the nausea. If it does not work after two doses, try the next indicated remedy.

Argentum Nitricum
Nervous nausea in anticipation of an event. Feels hurried, nervous, with diarrhoea.

Arsenicum Album
Nausea from nervous anticipation, with much thirst. He is so anxious he cannot bear the thought or sight of food. Loss of appetite, heart-burn.

Borax
Air sickness.

Cocculus
Nausea with faintness, after eating, after travel, from anxiety, exhaustion, travel motion.

Ipecacuanha
Nausea, persistent, constant, violent, with much empty belching, pale face, after eating or movement. The smell of food and tobacco smoke make him feel sick. Probably the basic first choice for nausea.

Nux Vomica
Nausea, constant after eating and drinking too much, in the morning, in bed, after breakfast, at the thought or smell of food.

Petroleum, Cocculus or *Tabacum*
Car sickness.

Pulsatilla
Nausea from rich fatty food, tobacco, with sensation of heavy weight in the stomach, some time after eating, with sour risings, no thirst.

Nelson's Homoeopathic Pharmacy sells an effective combination remedy called 'Travel Sickness Remedy'. Available from large pharmacies.

Nerves (Pre-Performance)

Argentum Nitricum
Nervous, impulsive and hurried. Cannot wait for the event to start and is very impatient. Cannot walk; wants to run. Believes that he will let people down and fail. Anxiety causes stiffness and tension. Often performs extremely well in preliminary rounds and seizes up in the final because it is a highly charged emotional occasion and he simply cannot cope with it. Mistakes creep into the performance because of the tension.

Nervous, possibly frequent, diarrhoea before the event. Cannot urinate because he fears diarrhoea. Short of breath, wants to take a deep breath, but this makes him worse. Bad dreams disturb sleep. Hurry, impatience and anxiety well hidden and under control. Does not want people to know he is nervous. You have to be very perceptive to recognise this.

Dosage: One Arg. Nit. 200c the evening before and another just before a major event. One at any time during an event to boost the nerves if he feels himself tensing up and his performance slipping.

Coca
The source of this remedy is the same as for the drug cocaine, which illegal users take to charge up their emotions and energy. The symptoms indicating homoeopathic Coca are as follows: The person suffers from stage fright. Nervous prostration alternates with exhilaration. Shy, nervous and withdrawn one minute, and a short time later cannot stop

talking. Avoids company, and is careless about appearance. Ecstatic and exalted, and becomes anxious with a feeling of pressure on the chest prevents proper breathing. Nausea with a headache, insomnia, frequent urination and fainting are other signs of someone who needs Coca.

The homoeopathic remedy Coca 200c does not contain any discernible cocaine, as the solution is more dilute than one drop in an Olympic swimming pool (see Chapter 3).
Dosage: Take one Coca 200c tablet before bed, and one hour before a match or performance.

Gelsemium

Shakes with fright. Sees the event as an ordeal and dreads it. Becomes paralysed with fear. Apathy and indifference about the outcome of the match or performance disguise his fright. Underneath he is terrified. Very drowsy but cannot sleep from the excitement of anticipation. Loss of sleep makes him want to withdraw. Loss of appetite and thirst. Wobbly knees. Loss of skills from muscle tension. Develops cold symptoms. Cannot relax. This person reacts in a way that is opposite to Arg. Nit. – the Gelsemium person slows down, whereas Arg. Nit. speeds up.
Dosage: One Gelsemium 200c the night before and one hour before the event.

You may consider combining Arg. Nit. and Gelsemium in one dose if you cannot differentiate between the two for an athlete or dancer who tends to succumb to nerves.

Lycopodium

This person needs a remedy because he loses self-confidence before any major event, but always performs well. His main problem is the inner conflict between natural anxiety and the knowledge that he can succeed. Normally confident and a bit superior and domineering, but wakes on the morning of an event full of anxiety, self doubt and anger. Nervousness makes him more domineering and superior before a match so that he upsets his team-mates. Weak stomach. Hungry, but can only eat very little before feeling very full. Noisy abdominal wind, distended when nervous. Anxious dreams keep him awake.
Dosage: One Lycopodium 200c the night before and on waking, and one immediately before the event, will relieve him and his colleagues of the effects of his nerves.

Nosebleed (see Epistaxis, page 193)

Period Problems and Amenorrhea Remedies

Intense physical activity and a restricted diet may lead to amenorrhea (cessation of periods). This in turn has been shown to increase the risk of osteoporosis. There are cases of athletes in their twenties and thirties with fractures regarded as osteoporotic. Gymnasts, especially girls who start serious training at a very young age, risk delaying the start of menstruation, and then experiencing irregular or absent periods. Cross and Boivin in a study of bone density in ballet dancers found that ballet dancers whose menses were few or none at all had significantly less dense bone in the lower spine. Dr Nicola Keay found that retired ballet dancers who had had the fewest periods or whose body weight had was furthest below the ideal for their height had the lowest spinal bone density, and that even when they resumed menstruating the bones had not recovered to the normal density for their age (*Dancing Times*, 9/95).

If an athlete's or dancer's periods are absent for six months or more they should see a specialist in case a gynaecological problem exists.

A qualified homoeopath will be able to prescribe a remedy to deal with all menstrual problems effectively, including amenorrhea. This could avoid the need to start taking some form of hormone replacement.

The following remedies may be found useful in restoring the periods, but, as just stated, should not be used to mask a condition that requires medical referral as well as advice from a qualified homoeopath.

Hypothalamus

This remedy may be useful when the amenorrhea is linked with physical overexertion, anorexia and psychological stress. The person is extremely sensitive, likeable and gentle by nature, given to alternating between smiles and tears. She is anxious, depressed, and mentally tired out with many thoughts cluttering her brain. Indecisive. Anxious at night. Dislikes raw foods such as salads, and sweets, appetite disorders, anorexia. Insomnia, or sudden overpowering need to sleep. Worse from cold. (Pulsatilla is better from cold fresh air.)
Dosage: One Hypothalamus 30c daily for three days.

Nux Moschata

Periods are irregular in time and quantity, or absent because of emotions and exertion. Hysterical by nature, given to fainting. Hates the thought of food, and can only digest highly seasoned food. Suffers from headaches. Great drowsiness. Listless and indifferent. Laughing and jesting. Forgets words when speaking. Sense of duality, thinks she is two persons.

Dosage: One Nux Moschata 30c daily for three days.

Pulsatilla

This is the first remedy to consider when periods are delayed in young girls who are mild, timid, emotional and tearful. Weeps easily, and craves sympathy. Loves company. Worse from eating rich foods, fats and ice cream, but also likes ice cream. Feels rejection and slight very deeply. Better in cool fresh air. Difficulty getting to sleep because she suddenly feels wide awake after performance and her thoughts go round and round. Often associated with digestive disorders.

Dosage: One Pulsatilla 30c daily for three days.

Sepia

This remedy is often effective for many menstrual problems including amenorrhea. Especially for women whose menstruation has never really settled down since puberty. Feels better from strenuous exercise and dancing. Voracious appetite or none at all. Nausea from thought of food. Desires chocolate, vinegar. Loathes fat. Aching and weakness in small of back, better from pressing against something hard.

Dosage: One Sepia 30c daily for three days.

There are many homoeopathic remedies that can work successfully for period pains, PMT and all the problems associated with the menstrual cycle. Menstrual problems may also respond to adjustments to diet.

Piles

Hamamelis

Large sore, bruised-feeling, bleeding piles that are worse in the open air and from sitting on hard cold surfaces.

Dosage: One Hamamelis 30c daily for three days. Hamamelis ointment may also help.

Nitric Acid

This remedy is not as bad as it sounds! The pain is burning, worse after stool, like a splinter in the anus with easy bleeding. The piles itch, but are worse from touch, and are also worse from warmth in bed. They are also worse in a cold damp atmosphere. They are agony when walking. *Dosage:* One Nitric Acid 30c daily for three days. Nitric Acid ointment may also help.

Paeonia

Biting itching in anus. Excruciating pain in the anus comes on after stool and continues for a long time. Must get up and walk about. Large ulcerated piles. Anal fissures or fistulas. Worse at night, from touch or pressure and after stool.
Dosage: One Paeonia 30c daily for three days. Also available as an ointment.

Sulphur-Iodum Ointment

This ointment is specifically useful for relieving the anal itching associated with piles.

Sciatica (see The Back and Neck, pages 162–72)

Sleeplessness (see Insomnia, pages 200–1)

Sore Throat

There are hundreds of homoeopathic remedies for sore throats. Here are a few first aid remedies for sore throats that I have found effective in the sports situation.

If the sore throat persists for more than a day or two you should consult a doctor or a qualified homoeopath.

Dosage: One tablet of the appropriate remedy should be taken in the 30c potency every hour for up to five doses. If the remedy does not alleviate the sore throat, try the next one indicated.

Aconite

Throat red, hot, dry, constricted, chokes on swallowing, brought on by exposure to cold air. The person seems frightened, looks pale and thinks he is dying.

Argentum Nitricum

Sensation of a splinter in the throat, with thick, tenacious mucus.

Belladonna
Very painful hot red and dry throat. Hot head and red face.

Causticum
Scraping, burning rawness, swallows continuously despite the pain. Hoarse.

Hepar Sulphuris
Sensation of splinter or fishbone with swollen ulcerated tonsils. Raw throat, pain extends into ears. Very sensitive to draughts. Coughing, turning the head, swallowing and cold drinks all hurt. Warm drinks make it better.

Lachesis
Left-sided pain extends into the ear, very painful to swallow but, strangely, food can be swallowed without pain. Throat very sensitive to external pressure and touch. Cannot bear clothing around throat.

Mercurius Corrosivus
Red, swollen throat, worse for the slightest pressure. Tonsils and all the glands around the throat swollen. Swallowing is very difficult.

Mercurius Solubilis
Sore, raw, burning, difficult, painful swallowing with pain into the ears. Offensive bad breath, indented tongue, much saliva.

Sunburn

Sunburn can be a serious and debilitating condition in athletes who overexpose themselves despite advice to the contrary. Belladonna 30c or Glonoine 30c may be given orally to counteract the effects of sunburn. See under 'Heatstroke' for details (pages 198–9).

Cantharis
For sunburn, if the pain is burning, smarting and cutting.
Dosage: One Cantharis 30c tablet dissolved in water for bathing the affected skin.

Urtica Urens Ointment
This ointment will relieve the pain of sunburn and prevent blistering, infection and pain.

Toothache

Mercurius Solubilis

Pain worse at night in bed, perhaps from an abscess, aggravated by draughts and cold air, tooth feels bruised, cheek swollen, pain spreads to ears, face and head, much saliva and very bad breath, with an indented tongue.

Dosage: One Mercurius 30c tablet dissolved in the mouth every hour for the pain, for five doses. Consult a dentist.

Tinea Cruris and Pedis

Itching in the groin, or between the toes, from a fungal infection from clothing or towels. Do not share towels after a shower or swim. The area should be kept clean and dry.

Calendula Cream

Applied as necessary to ease the itching.

Carbo Vegetabilis

Fiery, burning, itching between the toes. Oozing watery discharge. Foul foot sweat. The condition heals and breaks out again.

Dosage: One Carbo Veg. 30c daily for three days. Dissolve one tablet in water to make a lotion, and dab on the affected parts.

Graphites

Rawness in the folds of the skin, moist, burning, itching, exudes gluey yellow moisture. Worse from heat, warmth of bed, at night.

Dosage: One Graphites 30c tablet daily for four or five days. Also, dissolve one tablet in water and use as a lotion to bathe the affected parts.

Travel Sickness (see also **Nausea**, pages 202–3)

By sea. Cocculus 30c before sailing.

Car sickness. Petroleum, Cocculus, or Tabacum, or a combination of all three. One before a journey, and every two hours during the journey.

Air. Borax 30c. One before flying, and one every two hours during the flight.

Specific combination remedies for travel sickness are also available. See directions on the container.

Tummy Upsets (see Diarrhoea, pages 191–3)

Verrucas and Warts

Antimonium Crudum
Verrucas that burn and itch, especially at night in bed. Worse from pressure.
Dosage: One Ant. Crud. 30c daily for three days.

Calcarea Carbonica
Horny warts on hands and fingers. Verrucas. Tendency to ulcerate.
Dosage: One Calc. Carb. 30c daily for three days.

Causticum
Large and ragged, flat, hard, single, brittle warts near the fingernails. Bleed easily.
Dosage: One Causticum 30c daily for three days.

Thuja
Has the best reputation for eliminating verrucas and warts. Large, stinging, itching and bleeding. Scratching the warts make them bleed. Worse at night.
Dosage: Take one Thuja 30c and wait for results. As well as taking the tablet for verrucas, dissolve one tablet in water and bathe the feet in the solution daily.

Wounds

Choose the remedy according to the type of wound, bleeding etc.
Dosage: One tablet by mouth in the 6c potency.

Arnica
Wounds to muscles, head. With sore bruised pain. Bleeding. After surgery.

Calendula
Lacerations. More painful than expected. Also, make a lotion by dissolving one Calendula 30c tablet in water and bathing the wound with it.

210

Hepar Sulphuris
Inflamed, with redness around.

Hypericum
To nerve-rich parts. Crushed tissue. Teeth. Shooting pain after surgery and tooth extraction.

Ledum
Puncture wounds, especially to palm of hand or sole of foot.

Phosphorus
Bleeding freely with bright red blood, slow to clot.

Silica
Inflamed, with splinters and material inside. Troublesome scars from wounds. After surgery.

Staphysagria
After surgery, especially gynaecological. Wounds with clean sides, as from a knife.

Chapter 10

Descriptions of Remedies (Materia Medica)

Note: the symptoms listed in this chapter of materia medica are predominantly those that relate to the use of the remedies in treating sports, exercise and dance injuries. A fuller picture of these remedies can be obtained by reference to more complete materia medicas.

ABC

This 'combination remedy' is made from Aconite, Belladonna and Chamomilla, all in the 6c potency. See below for details of these remedies.

Complaints: Common cold.

General Uses: If taken at the first signs of a cold this remedy can hold it off for a few days or stop it altogether.

Aconite

The Monk's Hood, or Wolf's Bane, grows in moist pastures and wasteland all over Europe and Central Asia. The root contains a deadly poison, said to have been used by huntsmen to poison their arrows when hunting wolves.

The homoeopathic remedy is prepared from the green and flowering parts of the plant, chopped, pounded and the juice extracted. This is mixed with alcohol, diluted, succussed and potentised. In this way all the poisonous elements are removed, and only the healing properties retained.

Causation: Exposure to cold. Fright.

Worse: Chill. Shock. Cold. Night.

Better: Rest.

Complaints: Cough. Colds. Fright. Accidents.

212

General Uses: For a short, dry, painful barking cough brought on suddenly by exposure to dry cold conditions or being chilled. It is worse in the evening or at night, and aggravated by breathing, smoking and drinking. It should be the first remedy to try after exposure to chill. He grasps his throat when he coughs. Very anxious and restless. Pale, frightened face.

Shock following injuries or accident when the person is thoroughly frightened. Extremely fearful and anxious.

Mental/Emotional: Great anxiety, agonising fear and restlessness. Sleep disturbed by re-enacting the trauma. Fears he will die.

Aesculus Hippocastanum

The horse chestnut.

Worse: Winter. Lying, stooping, standing. Cold air.

Better: Keeping moving.

Complaints: Backache in sacrum.

Back: Constant ache in the sacrum, much worse from bending forward and walking. It is almost impossible to rise after sitting. The sacrum feels bruised and weak. The pain may strike suddenly and prevents him from working or training. Worse on waking in the morning.

Mental: Very irritable. Confused. Gloomy.

Allium Cepa

The common red onion has been renowned among country people for a very long time for its healing properties. It is said to purify the blood and clear the intestines of worms. The homoeopathic remedy is made from the whole bulb, gathered in July or August, chopped and pounded to a pulp before the juice is extracted and succussed.

Worse: In a warm room. Wet feet.

Better: Cool open air.

Complaints: Colds. Hay fever.

General Uses: Cold that comes on after exposure to biting cold damp wind. There is a constant drip of watery copious discharge, and the nose is red and raw. Hot and thirsty. Worse in the evening and indoors. Hay fever. The eyes stream with water, but they are not sore. The nose streams with water, and becomes very sore. There is frequent violent sneezing and a raw sore throat. It is worse in spring and August, and in a warm room.

Alumina

The metal. The remedy is made by trituration.

Worse: Waking. Warm dry weather. Exercise. On alternate days.

Better: Cold bathing. Gentle exertion.

Complaints: Carpal tunnel syndrome.

Upper Limbs: This remedy has the unusual symptom that the person feels as if a red hot needle is being inserted into the finger. The fingers are heavy, as if paralysed, with pins and needles after going to sleep. Loss of coordination. Worse in a warm room and after a warm bath. The condition may resolve without reason, and then return later.

Mental: A hasty person for whom time passes too slowly. Grumpy on waking. Becomes depressed, and moans about things.

Anacardium Orientale

Commonly known as the Marking Nut because of the black juice extracted from it. Related to the cashew. Grows in the East Indies. The remedy is made by powdering and triturating the layer between the shell and the nut itself.

Worse: Physical and mental exertion. Evening.

Better: Eating. In the sun.

General Uses: Muscle pains, tears, cramps, trembling, almost paralysis. Muscles tear easily although what he suspects, for example, to be a hamstring tear usually turns out to be a cramp.

Mental/Emotional: Exaggerates the effects of injury. Full of conflict. Seems to be two people and cannot decide which to be. One part is determined to succeed with a fixed idea of objectives. The other lacks confidence and predicts difficulties. Becomes ill-tempered, exhausted and paralysed with tiredness. Lacks the power to perform.

Angustura Vera

Derived from the bark of the South American plant, *Galipea cusparia*, as used for bitters.

Worse: Rest, exertion, pressure, putting foot down.

Better: Stretching, cold applications.

Complaints: Soreness and pain in joints of the foot and medial side of ankle when walking or standing. Lameness.

General Uses: Sensation of weakness and stiffness, tension in muscles when walking, cracking of joints, twitching and jerking of muscles.

Upper limbs: Arms tired and heavy, stiffness of elbow.

Lower limbs: Pain in ankles when walking, sore, bruised pain in heel, sole and joints of foot, sensation of blunt body under foot, worse from pressure.

Mental/Emotional: Timid, lacks self-confidence, takes offence, excited and vivacious in the afternoon.

Apis Mellifica

Derived from the honey bee, the remedy has the burning, stinging, smarting of the bee sting itself among its symptoms.

Worse: Heat in any form. Touch and pressure.

Better: Cool air and bathing.

Complaints: Carpal tunnel syndrome.

Upper Limbs: Numbness of tips of fingers with stinging pains that come on extremely suddenly. He may believe he has been stung. Burning and soreness are present. The fingers may be red, swollen and itching. Palms hot and swollen. They are worse from touch. He wants to keep cool, and hates heat. Awkward, and drops things. Trembling. In the same way as Arnica, he says there is nothing wrong and is indifferent to his condition.

Argentum Nitricum

Silver nitrate is used in the manufacture of photographic film and mirrors, and has been used in solution as a fungicide. The homoeopathic remedy is made from the dissolved crystals.

Worse: Anxiety. Emotions. Indoors, especially in tightly enclosed spaces.

Better: Cool open air.

Complaints: Nerves and anxiety. Sore throat.

General Uses: Frequent nervous diarrhoea before an event. Cannot urinate because he fears involuntary diarrhoea. Short of breath, wants to take a deep breath, but this makes him worse. Sore throat with feeling of splinter in it, worse swallowing. Thick sticky mucus in throat makes him hawk and swallow.

Mental/Emotional: Nervous, impulsive and hurried. Very impatient. Very hurried. Has to run. Cannot walk. Believes he will let people down and fail. Very anxious. Stiffens up and becomes tense. Cannot relax. Loses form. Cannot cope with a highly charged emotional occasion. Dreams disturb sleep. Hurry, impatience and anxiety are well hidden.

Arnica Montana

This remedy is made from a common alpine plant. Its German name is 'Fallkraut', which implies that it cures the effects of falls. And it does!

More than any other remedy, Arnica is the treatment for trauma in all varieties and its effects, whether recent or remote. It prevents the overreaction of the vascular system to traumatic injury from blows and falls. Prevents and reduces the effects of shock. Limits extravasation into joint capsules, and reduces the subsequent atrophy of surrounding muscles.

Arnica should be the first remedy to be given in every case of traumatic injury – without fail. Even the smallest blow or accident will respond. It controls bleeding, reduces swelling and prevents pus forming. In this way it promotes speedy recovery, and should be in every first aid kit and in every home.

Causation: Trauma – accidents, falls, blows, strains, sprains, twisting, bruising, bleeding, blows to the head, overexertion and unaccustomed exercise. Muscle strains and tears. Massage and manipulation.

Worse: Touch, jarring, exertion, damp, cold, the threat of further injury, or even treatment.

Better: Lying with the head lower than the feet. Warmth.

Complaints: Restlessness. Shock. Muscles very sore and painful, feels bruised all over. Cannot sleep because the bed feels too hard. Bruising, swelling, bleeding. He avoids exertion of any kind. Dazed, cold, shaking, fainting, confused after injury. Nausea, headache, following injury. Bleeding, open wounds which may become infected. Arnica given orally will stop bleeding internally and externally and prevent infection.

General Uses: Use Arnica after every trauma, even the slightest, to prevent shock, short and long-term effects of injury and to speed recovery. Prevents the development of haematoma in large muscles after blows or tears, and assist the dispersal of those haematomae without the development of intramuscular calcification. Compound and closed fractures. Do not forget Arnica for the after-effects of shocks to the system, such as marathon running, long-distance air travel or infections such as flu. It is excellent for helping recovery from operations, and even childbirth. Use after head injuries and concussion.

Upper limbs: Elbows and shoulders feel dislocated, bruised and sore. Bruising and swelling of muscles and joints. Stiffness and weariness of arms and shoulders after trauma or unaccustomed exertion. Direct blows to and tears in the biceps and other muscles. Dislocation of shoulder and elbow; fractures of all bones, especially compound fractures of the long bones. Trauma to the hand, fingers and wrist.

Lower limbs: Painful paralytic weakness of hips and knees. Soreness in the legs and painful swelling of the knee. Stiffness and weariness of legs after unaccustomed exertion. Compound and closed fractures. Fractures of all kinds. Blows or tears to large muscles, especially if there is risk of haematoma. To assist dispersal of haematoma. Trauma of any kind resulting in bruising, haematoma, shock. Immediately following sprains and strains to ligaments, meniscus tears, traumatic derangement of hip, knee and ankle joints. Helps to prevent bleeding and reduce effusion.

Back: Bruised pains in back, great soreness, cervical vertebrae tender and weak. Difficult to hold the head up, wants to lean head back.

Mental/Emotional: Says that he is OK, and does not want treatment. When asked, he says, 'I'm fine, just leave me alone,' because he fears treatment may hurt more. Fears touch, shies away from contact with

217

others, or from further injury. Sleep difficult because the bed is too hard, and he has anxious dreams.

Arsenicum Album

This remedy is derived from an oxide of arsenic. The poison has been used as a tonic by many people, and as a stimulant for animals. The signs of poisoning by arsenic are nausea, vomiting, diarrhoea and even paralysis. The homoeopathic remedy is prepared by roasting the arsenides of iron, nickel and cobalt, grinding up the residue and potentising this by trituration and succussion.

It is one of the great polychrests of the homoeopathic materia medica and has uses for most disease conditions and pathologies.

Causation: Chills, bad food, travel. Muscle tears, trauma, overuse.

Worse: Cold, cold air, cold bathing, cold food, contaminated food or drink. Exertion, lying on affected part. After midnight, every two weeks. At 2 a.m.

Better: Heat, hot applications, bathing, food. Demands cold drinks for upset stomach. Walking about in the open air.

Complaints: Sickness and diarrhoea from food poisoning. Carpal tunnel syndrome, hamstring tears, ankle conditions, foot pain, black toenail.

General Uses: More affected by the injury or condition than its seriousness would suggest. Prostrated and very weak. Pains burn like fire, hot needles or wire, but are relieved by heat. Sudden great weakness. Very restless.

Upper limbs: Tingling and burning in the fingers, which cannot be extended. Drawing pain from wrist to elbow.

Lower limbs: Blue, discoloured toenails. Burning pain in balls of feet. Feet weak, weary and numb. Sore pain in ankles. Restless feet. Burning pain in hamstring which feels tightly contracted. Stiffness and lameness with pain behind the thigh, cannot extend the knee. Burning pain, but heat relieves it. Moves his feet constantly. Is much worse from cold in any form.

Back: Weak lumbar region, bruised pain in small of back. Stiffness from coccyx to neck.

Mental/Emotional: Seeks medical opinions and help from many sources. Very sensitive, fastidious, irritable and careful with money.

Security-conscious, checks he has locked things. Believes he cannot recover, and forecasts all kinds of disaster as a result of his injury. Very restless, moves from place to place but cannot rest. Likes company, and dislikes being alone. Imagines all sorts of disasters when alone. Selfish. Feels he wants to die.

Aurum Metallicum

This remedy is made from gold, by trituration. It is another of the polychrests of the homoeopathic materia medica.

The deep bone pains of Aurum may arise frequently when treating the long-term effects of sports injuries.

Causation: Effects of fright, grief or anger. Frightening trauma.

Worse: Emotional upset, guilt, cold weather, winter, at night.

Better: Walking in the open air, moonlight, warmth, music.

Complaints: Foot pain. Bone pains.

General Uses: Pain, as if bruised, felt deep in the bones.

Upper limbs: Boring pains in the left shoulder. Cramp-like acute drawing pains in the palms and fingers.

Lower limbs: Drawing pains, cramping, in the bones and joints of the toes.

Back: Violent back pains in the morning.

Mental/Emotional: Very depressed, and suicidal. Feels very strong guilt about injury, as if he had committed a crime. Angry and violently quarrelsome.

Badiaga

The freshwater sponge.

Worse: Cold, pressure, touch.

Better: Heat.

Complaints: Bruised, sore heels, epiphysitis of calcaneum.

Lower limbs: Bruised heel, very sore, worse from pressure, he does not want to put it to the ground. Skin soreness, epiphysitis. Anterior muscles of leg sore, as if beaten.

Baryta Carbonica

Barium carbonate.

Worse: Lying on painful side, cold damp, heat of sun or stove.

Better: Cold food, wrapping up warmly, when alone.

Complaints: Common cold, exhaustion, bursitis in knee, loss of confidence.

Lower limbs: Pain in the knees when kneeling.

Mental/Emotional: Shy, timid, mistrustful, loses self-confidence. Especially among strangers. Thinks he is being laughed at and made fun of. Avoids company and does not want to socialise. Loses self-confidence. Very childish in behaviour. This sometimes gets him into trouble. Not to be confused with nervousness and anxiety before an event, this person is fundamentally and childishly shy and nervous. Can sometimes react violently, as a child may do.

Belladonna

The common name for Belladonna is Deadly Nightshade, one of the best known of British poisonous plants. Its bright red berries have caused many accidental poisonings amongst children. It is becoming more rare in Britain but still grows in some woody and shady places. Even handling the leaves is dangerous.

The symptoms of poisoning by Belladonna have given the homoeopath a guide to conditions that it will cure – dry mouth, red hot fever, sore throat, nausea and dizziness.

The homoeopathic remedy is made from the entire plant, including the flowers, chopped and pounded, and the juice expressed. This is mixed with alcohol, allowed to stand for eight days, and then potentised.

Causation: Exposure to the sun. Cold dry wind. Getting the head wet.

Worse: Heat of sun, cold, motion.

Better: Rest in the shade, in a dark room, bending backward.

Complaints: Colds. Sore throat. Sunstroke. Headache.

General Uses: Very painful, hot, red and dry throat brought on after too much sun, or exposure to cold. Swallowing very difficult, yet has to swallow all the time. Can only swallow very small sips of water. Has to bend forward to swallow. Headache from the sun, throbbing, hammering, in the temples or back of head, worse from motion, jarring, sunlight. Better from lying in a dark room. Hot red face.

Mental/Emotional: Angry, anxious, delirious, confused, excitable. Restless, tosses and turns. Very sensitive to light, noise, and the slightest jarring.

Bellis Perennis

The common daisy is also known as Wound Wort, and, like Arnica, is a great traumatic remedy. It was used by country people as a cure for wounds. The fresh flowering plant is chopped and crushed, and the juice mixed with alcohol. It stands for eight days before being filtered and potentised.

Causation: Blows and injuries, cooling or wetting when overheated.

Worse: Injuries, sprains, touch, cold baths, becoming chilled after being hot, surgical operations.

Better: Continued motion, cold applications.

Complaints: Bruises to soft tissue, sore, bruised muscles, injuries to male and female genitalia and breasts. Abdominal bruising.

General Uses: Bellis may be useful if Arnica does not seem to have worked. This remedy has a special affinity for soft tissue injuries, and haemorrhages following blows to parts consisting of such sensitive tissue. The pains may be throbbing, aching or squeezing, and are so unbearable they drive one to distraction.

Lower limbs: Deep intense bruised pain in the ankle which feels as if it has an elastic bandage around it. Calf muscle tears, if Arnica does not relieve the pain, and the pain is deep in the muscle and unbearable. Collateral ligament injuries. The knee feels better from heat and hot applications. The pain and bruising is deeper than in Arnica and may be felt down the front of the thigh. Dead leg from blow to quadriceps.

Mental/Emotional: In contrast to Arnica, the Bellis person tells you he is injured and needs help, does not like the idea of ice if he is still hot from activity but finds that the ice treatment is very effective and relieves the pain. Moves impulsively.

Berberis

The barberry is a native British plant that grows on heaths and mountains. The remedy is made from a tincture of the bark of the root.

Worse: Motion, jarring, rising from sitting, standing.

Complaints: Lower back pain. Kidney conditions.

Back: Backache with severe prostration and crushing, stitching, paralysing pain in lumbar region. Worse sitting and lying, rising from a seat, standing and motion. The pain radiates down the front of the thighs. Cannot walk even a short distance.

Mental/Emotional: Apathetic and indifferent.

Borax

Borax is a white mineral found in Tibet, Peru and other mountain areas. It is used industrially in many manufacturing processes, including glass, porcelain and paper. The homoeopathic remedy is prepared from dissolving out the borax from a compound of boracic acid and sodium carbonate.

Worse: Downward and upward motion. Sudden noises.

Complaints: Fear of flying. Motion sickness from flying.

Generals: Upward and downward motion of flying. Nausea, pain in stomach. Distension, belching. Vertigo. Ears feel closed up. Ear pain after flying. Abdominal wind.

Mental/Emotional: Nervous, anxious, irritable, fidgety, starts or frightened by sudden noise. Fear of flying. Wakes at 4 a.m. with fear of flying. Sleeps badly during flight.

Bryonia Alba

The White Bryony, or wild hop, is a climbing perennial that grows wild in woods and vineyards in southern Britain and central and southern Europe. It has bright green leaves and black berries. The common hedgerow plant, also called white bryony, is *Bryonia doica*, and has red berries. The plant has long been used as a herbal remedy for coughs. The homoeopathic remedy is made from juice from the pulp of the fresh root.

Causation: Anger, fright, cold winds, trauma.

Worse: The least motion, rising, stooping, coughing, exertion, deep breathing, hot weather, getting hot, touch, early morning, 9 p.m.

Better: Pressure, lying on painful part, bandaging, cool open air, quiet, cloudy damp days, heat to inflamed part, cold drinks.

Complaints: All conditions and injuries when the least movement is painful; stress fractures, foot pains, osteoarthritis, ankle sprains, knee conditions, after knee surgery, shoulder injuries, carpal tunnel syndrome and lower back pain may all be helped by this remedy if the symptoms fit. Coughs, nosebleeds, colds, flu.

General Uses: Osteoarthritis, if the pain is aggravated by even the smallest movement, and increases with exercise and exertion. Intense pain and fatigue make him want to lie in one position only and not move a finger. Oversensitive to anything that requires effort or motion, avoids conversation. Weak and tired feeling in the limbs, hot red swelling of joints, very sensitive to touch. Cough worse in the evening and lying down. Holds the chest when coughing. Stitching pains. May be required when Arnica does not seem to work. The person is reluctant to exercise even when the lower leg is still immobilised in a cast. Moving eyelids and eyes painful. Any movement, even the least, and of any part makes this person feel bad.

Upper limbs: The arm and shoulder feel too weak to move. Raising the arm is very painful and makes him feel bad. The joint feels swollen and hot. The pain is burning and tearing, and the shoulder feels pulled out of place. Acromioclavicular sprain. Dislocation of the elbow when any movement is very painful. Pins and needles in the fingers, following numbness. Carpal tunnel syndrome. There is stitching pain with hot red swelling around the finger joints. Moving the fingers painful. Hand is weak and cannot grip.

Lower limbs: Stress fractures of the metatarsals when pain increases with activity or movement. Hallux rigidus when any movement is painful. Pain in the feet like pins and needles. They are swollen and hot. The soles are painful as soon as they touch the ground, but are better when pressure is put on them. Then they are sore again when lifted. Heat is unbearable. Every and any movement is painful. Ankle sprains; even the least movement is avoided. The swelling may be red, hot and painful to touch, but, strangely, better when it is pressed or held.

Fractures. Anterior knee pain and collateral ligament injuries with hot red swelling around the patella. Better from pressure on the knee, likes to have it bound up tightly and kept cool. The knee feels weak and bends under him. After knee surgery to promote movement and exercise.

Back: Back pain. Stitching pain in the small of the back that is worse from any movement. The pain is worse from turning and walking. Stiffness too, prevents stooping.

Mental/Emotional: Fears to move, talk or even breathe because of the possibility of pain. Look out for the mental symptoms that the person does not say much, wants to be left alone and may want to go home before treatment is over or even before it begins. Irritable and angry.

Calcarea Carbonica

Calcium carbonate, as limestone, is found everywhere in the world. It has been formed from the fossilised shells of sea creatures. Calc. Carb., the homoeopathic remedy, is made from the pure white layer found between the interior and exterior layers of the oyster shell. This is ground to a powder and triturated.

Causation: Overlifting, strains, injury to lower spine, fright, cold moist winds, immersion in cold water, floods. Overexertion.

Worse: Exertion, cold bathing, cold raw air, standing.

Better: Lying down, heat, being constipated.

Complaints: Cramping pains in back and joints, weak, frequently spraining ankles, Achilles tendon tears. Knee, collateral ligament, and surgery. Inguinal pain. Carpal tunnel syndrome. Lower back injuries. Frequent colds. Slow mending bones after a fracture.

General Uses: Sluggish temperament with fair skin. Slumps, avoids exertion. Flabby. Lazy about training, or does just enough. Lack endurance. Disappointing performance, below potential. Craves boiled eggs, and dislikes coffee and meat. Sweats easily about the head and neck. Muscles strain and atrophy easily. Injuries and complaints often follow cold and damp conditions, or playing in wet cold weather and getting heated. Stitching inguinal pains the result of a sprain following physical exertion. This remedy has an affinity with the inguinal glands and could be effective if infection is a suspected cause of the pain. Painful haemorrhoids worse when walking and better for sitting. Use Calc. Carb. if Symphytum is not effective in healing broken bones.

Upper limbs: Tearing, neuralgic pain in the fingers. He will have cold, flabby, damp hands. His fingers are numb when gripping, and are stiff and immobile. Cramps at night, arthritic pain, and swelling. Worse from cold air, bathing and exertion. Weak wrists that sprain easily in heavily built, overweight, flabby, fair children, young people and adults.

Lower limbs: Weak ankles that turn over too easily in heavily built, overweight, flabby, fair children, young people and adults. Tearing pain in tendons. Cold damp feet, cramps at night, arthritic pain, and swelling in the knee of the injured limb. This remedy can be useful when the knee condition is generated by pronation of the feet from weak ankles. Pain worse when rising from a seat and when sitting. Weakness and trembling in the limb. Feet cold and flabby. The knee will be worse from bandaging or support. The knee continues to swell following exertion some time after the injury, when the athlete or dancer has resumed active exercise.

Back: This tends to be the weightlifter's back remedy. Problems from overlifting. The back feels sprained and he cannot get up from a seat. Cannot sit up straight. Slumps in a seat. Feeling of dislocation in the sacroiliac and looseness in the vertebrae. Back is painful on pressure (compare with Sepia). Shooting pains in the back that are worse at night, and when riding in a car or bus. It hurts to breathe.

Mental/Emotional: Often avoids training, but once a routine is established works very hard at it. Dislikes change and can be obstinate and headstrong. Worries that friends think him stupid. Depressed and sad about the injury. Expresses doubts about recovery, and becomes depressed about it. Naturally flabby and inclined to put on weight easily, but works hard at fitness.

Calcarea Fluorica

Fluorspar, fluoride of lime, occurs worldwide and is found in the surface of bones, the enamel of teeth and elastic tissue. Its crystals are usually violet-coloured and emit blue light under ultraviolet.

This Schüssler tissue salt is especially related to bone and bony conditions. As such it is used for tooth decay, relaxing elastic tissue and glands, and dispersing bony growths. Calc. Fluor. may be needed if Rhus Tox. seems not to have worked.

Worse: Beginning of motion, cold, wet, sprains, changing weather.

Better: Continued motion, warm applications, heat, rubbing.

Complaints: Calcification and ossification in ligaments and tendons. Worn out, flabby and lax tissues. General stiffness. Tooth decay. Indurations. Weakness in the morning.

General Uses: Loose, decaying, crumbling teeth. Promotes the recovery of damaged fibrous tissue. Indurations and swellings around tendons. It can arrest the development of bony growths and reduce exostoses.

Lower limbs: This a very specific remedy for pain and tenderness over the medial collateral ligament associated with calcification and possibly ossification in the ligament. It is sometimes needed following repeated medial ligament sprains or haematoma from direct blows. The pain is worse after rest and relieved by moving a little, not as much as Rhus Tox., and by warm applications.

Back: Pains in the lower back that are worse on first moving and better from continued motion.

Calendula

The marigold, from which this remedy is made, is an annual flowering plant with tall, deep orange flowers. Cooks and herbalists have used it for hundreds of years as a salad and as a highly respected healer of diseases of the skin.

The homoeopathic remedy is made from the leaves, flowers and buds. They are pulped, the expressed juice mixed with alcohol and the solution succussed.

It is available as a cream, ointment or lotion from homoeopathic pharmacies, and for oral consumption in tablet form. I find that the cream is the most effective for skin conditions.

Causation: Laceration, bruising, burns, abrasion, falls and blows, infections and bites.

Complaints: Open, torn, cut, lacerated, ragged or suppurating wounds. Dry, itching, sore skin. Burns. Whenever the pain is more than should be expected for the condition or injury.

General Uses: Promotes healing of cuts and lacerations. Prevents infection.

Cantharis

This remedy is derived from the 'Spanish fly'. The insect has a reputation as an aphrodisiac because of its irritating effect on the kidneys and urinary tract. This probably makes the victim more conscious of his or her genitalia, and reputedly drives them into a sexual frenzy.

To make the homoeopathic remedy the flies are killed by steaming, then dried, crushed and ground into a powder with lactose sugar. Dilution and potentisation proceed as usual.

Worse: Urinating, touch, coffee.

Better: Warmth, rest, rubbing.

Complaints: Blisters, sunburn, burns of all sorts, continuous erections (priapism).

General Uses: Smarting, sore, burning pains

Carcinosin

Carcinosin is made from cancerous tissue and has become one of the well-used modern remedies. (In homoeopathic terms it is a 'nosode' – i.e. a remedy made from diseased tissue.) In this book it is recommended almost specifically for dancers who suffer from the long-term build-up of anxiety and stress.

Causation: Prolonged stress.

Better: Open air.

Worse: Extreme weather. Strenuous exercise

Complaints: Uncontrollable nervousness, stage fright, anticipation.

Mental/Emotional: Anxiety and fear of what may happen and what may go wrong. Passionately emotional people who overextend themselves. Very sympathetic to the needs of others. Very conscientious towards the company and friends. Loves to travel. Deep guilt if injured. Loves dancing and music almost obsessively. Very ambitious, perhaps as the result of parental ambition for them. Insomnia. Very badly affected by criticism, reprimand or contradiction. Excited by thunderstorms. Very fastidious about appearance, punctuality, cleanliness and possessions, even more so than Arsenicum. Anxiety that increases with each performance, despite experience. It is as if she believes that failure is certain after a set number of performances. Convinced she will fail, yet fears failure. Conscious of the effort and cost of her training and of owing a debt for that to others. Fear of cancer. Superstitious.

Causticum

Causticum, or potassium hydrate, is a compound made first by Hahnemann by mixing slaked lime (calcium hydroxide) with bisulphate of potash.

Causation: Burns or scalds, fright, grief or sorrow, insomnia.

Worse: Dry, cold winds, exertion, change of weather, travelling, 3–4 a.m., evenings.

Better: Damp weather, cold drinks, warmth, in bed, washing.

Complaints: Weak ankles. Cracking joints. Cramps. Achilles tendon tears. Shin splints. Stress fractures. Osgood-Schlatter disease. Posterior knee pain. Restlessness. Dislocations. Scraping, burning sore throat with hoarseness. Continuous swallowing as if to keep the throat clear. Swallows the wrong way and saliva comes through nose.

General Uses: Burns that itch painfully.

Upper Limbs: Dislocated shoulder. Paralysis in the arm, and deltoid. Cannot raise arm to head. Pain is tearing, rheumatic and raw. Tries to stretch, bend or crack the joints. Shoulder feels dislocated and 'paralysed.' Without a lot of encouragement this patient is really going to have a paralysed shoulder.

Lower Limbs: Weak ankles, walking is unsteady. Tearing rheumatic pain in the joint. Tendons and ligaments feel contracted, preventing movement. Cracking in the joint. Cramps in the foot and calf. Legs are restless at night. Pain like electric shocks in leg. Stiffness worse from sitting and relieved by walking. Severe tearing, rheumatic pain in the region and the Achilles tendon feels contracted. The joint may be burning, and deformed.

Tearing, rheumatic, burning anterior leg pain. Like an electric shock in the leg. Pain is much worse in the morning in bed, but better when he is warm in bed at night. The pain is much worse from getting cold, or having ice treatment. Tension in the knee, especially when descending. Stiffness in the hollow of the knee.

Back: Stiff neck, cannot move the head. Cramps in lumbar region and buttocks.

Mental/Emotional: Anxious and depressed, sensitive and guilty about being injured. Feels he has let down the team. Mentally tired and worried about the future. After loss or grief in the past. Very sensitive to the feelings of others, and very sympathetic. Inclined to take up causes. Will ask others about their problems rather than have his own dealt with. Overworked and exhausted from caring for others, or for animals.

Chelidonium

The English common name for *Chelidonium majus* is Greater Celandine. It grows in rather wet places in Britain and Europe. Under the 'Doctrine of Signatures' the ancients used the plant as a remedy for jaundice, because it stains the skin a deep yellow colour. Homoeopathically it is best known as a liver remedy, and works mainly on the right side of the body.

The juice of the whole flowering plant is used, diluted with alcohol and succussed.

Worse: Motion, 4 a.m. and 4 p.m., touch, change of weather.

Better: Eating hot food, hot bath, lying on abdomen.

Complaints: Right-sided. Ankle sprains, fractures and injuries. Anterior knee pain, collateral ligament injuries. Rotator cuff injuries, acromio-clavicular pain,

General Uses: Although touch makes it worse, pressure may relieve the pain. Chelidonium is similar to Bryonia in that movement is painful, but Chelidonium's stiffness is more rigid, and the muscles are more in spasm. Bryonia is afraid to move; Chelidonium cannot move. If Bryonia does not work on an injured right shoulder, try Chelidonium.

Upper limbs: A painful right shoulder makes him unable to use his arm. The least touch is exceedingly painful, as is abduction. Tearing, neuralgic and rheumatic pain. The arm feels heavy, stiff and flabby and there may be trembling. Pain extends from the shoulder to under the scapula, and there may be a stiff neck. Pain under the scapula on moving the arm and breathing.

Lower limbs: The ankle, usually the right, is very stiff and burning. The stiffness is worse from moving but better after warm bathing. The pain is worse at 4 p.m. and 4 a.m. Pain, burning, and stiffness in the right knee, especially in the patellar tendon. The knee is very sore to touch, and the limb feels heavy and paralysed. Continuing stiffness and swelling in the right knee after exertion.

Mental/Emotional: Restless, depressed and anxious as if he had done something wrong. Lethargic and drowsy but has trouble sleeping and wakes at 4 a.m. Anxious, despondent and guilty about being injured. Lethargic in approach to training and playing, and inclined to be 'liverish' in the morning.

China

Peruvian bark, or *Cinchona officinalis*, was the first substance proved by Hahnemann. It is the main source of quinine, and was used from the middle of the 17th century onwards to treat malaria, or 'the ague' as it was then known.

The bark is dried and powdered, mixed with alcohol, left to stand for eight days, and the liquor strained and filtered before succussion.

Causation: Eating contaminated fruit, fish or meat. Drinking contaminated water.

Worse: After eating, exertion.

Better: Bending double, tight clothing.

Complaint: Diarrhoea.

Generals: Diarrhoea, painless, in hot weather. Dark, watery, foul stools consisting mainly of undigested food. Preceded by flatulent bloating and colic. Caused by fruit, milk, beer, bad fish, meat or water. Drenching cold sweats at stool. Terrible weakness. Better after a short rest. Insomnia from fantasies.

Mental/Emotional: Apathetic, depressed, averse to training, playing or exertion. Indifferent to everything, or else very touchy, irritable and sensitive.

Coca

Coca leaves have been chewed for centuries by the natives of upland Peru and Patagonia to enable them to work at high altitudes. Latterly the tree has become infamous as the source of cocaine. The homoeopathic remedy is so dilute that there is absolutely none of the drug remaining in the solution. It is legal and safe to use.

Causation: Altitude, long flights.

Worse: High altitude, mental exertion, cold, walking, exertion.

Better: Rapid motion, after sunset, open air, lying on abdomen.

Complaints: Altitude. Shortage of breath, dizziness, weakness and exhaustion. Pre-match nerves. Exhaustion and fatigue.

General Uses: Effects of altitude. Shortage of breath, breathing becomes fast and difficult, especially in older athletes. Short hacking cough generated by tickling and irritation in the larynx. Paroxysmal and debilitating cough. The person can faint from weakness. Yellow phlegm. Headache in the forehead or occiput, or both, aggravated by coughing. Vertigo, violent palpitations, nosebleeds, nausea and hoarseness. Sleep is disturbed and restless, with many dreams. One of the strange effects of altitude is that people can become elated and euphoric, which are mental symptoms of Coca. Another effect of altitude is called 'glacier lassitude'. Prostration is also one of the symptoms of Coca. This remedy counteracts the effects of long periods at an altitude of between 5,000 ft and 8,000 ft, which the cabin pressurisation of most commercial aircraft produces. It can help a person to sleep during a long flight, and to recover from jet lag.

Lower limbs: Swelling of ankles, restless legs after a long flight.

Mental/Emotional: Prostration alternates with exhilaration, timid, bashful, hides away, blissful daydreams, neglects personal appearance. Ecstatic and exalted, and then becomes anxious with a feeling of pressure on his chest.

Cocculus Indicus

This plant is called Indian Berry and grows in Asia. It is also called the 'Fish Berry' because its seeds were scattered on water to stun fish. The seeds have been used by robbers to stupefy their victims. The homoeopathic remedy is made by mixing the seeds with alcohol and heating gently for twenty-four hours. The liquor is strained and succussed.

Worse: Motion of boats, cars, trains, buses. Cold, open air.

Better: Sitting. Lying on side.

Complaints: Travel sickness. Nausea. Headache. Exhaustion.

Generals: Exhaustion and complaints from travel. Nausea with faintness, after eating. Lost appetite, from anxiety, exhaustion, travel motion. Headache with nausea, especially when travelling by boat or car.

Coffea Cruda

Coffee is said to counter the effects of wine. The opposite is also true; a glass of wine after drinking too much coffee will encourage a person to sleep. Tea and beer can have similar effects on each other. Although many people find that too much coffee excites them too much to sleep, the homoeopathic remedy is excellent at helping people to sleep when they feel excited. This remedy is made from the unroasted coffee bean.

Causation: Overexcitement. Great pleasure. Success. Good news. Overtiredness. Long journeys.

Worse: Noise, touch, open air, mental exertion, emotions, alcohol, narcotics, night.

Better: Lying, sleep, warmth.

Complaints: Insomnia.

General Uses: For the person who cannot sleep from excitement, over-tiredness, after a long journey, anticipation of the next day's event, receiving good news or feelings of pleasure after a successful day. Hearing every sound, becomes irritable from wakefulness.

Colchicum Autumnale

This plant resembles the crocus but blooms in the autumn, which is the reason for its common name of Autumn Crocus. It is, however, a type of lily and is very poisonous. It has been used as a herbal remedy for gout and rheumatism since the 13th century. One early herbalist noted that it also had the ability to cause gout, which appears to support the theory of homoeopathy that 'like cures like'. The homoeopathic reme-dy is prepared from the fresh bulb, before flowering. It is chopped and crushed, the extracted juice mixed with alcohol and succussed.

Worse: Motion, touch, cold damp weather, at night.

Better: Warmth, rest.

Complaint: Gout.

Lower limbs: Gout. Tearing pain in toe and foot, Cannot bear to have foot touched. Oedematous swelling of affected joint. Worse for the slightest movement, cold, and at night.

Mental/Emotional: Depressed, irritable, sensitive to pain and disturbance. Sits very still without moving. Fears the slightest touch.

Colocynthis

This plant grows in hot sandy places all over the world, and is better known as Squirting Cucumber. Its yellow fruits are very poisonous, and have been used as purgatives since ancient times. The Old Testament prophet Elisha miraculously turned the fruit into nutritious food during a famine. The homoeopathic remedy is prepared from the fruit. This is powdered, soaked in alcohol, and macerated. The liquid is then extracted and succussed.

Worse: At night, in bed.

Better: Hard pressure. Bending double.

Complaints: Colic. Diarrhoea. Sciatica.

General: Dysentery and diarrhoea. Violent, cutting, gripping, clutching, colicky pains that come in waves across abdomen. Watery, yellow, shreddy, painful stools squirt out. Following the least food or drink.

Lower limbs: Sudden, terrible, cramping, tearing, neuralgic pain down the sciatic nerve that makes the person cry out. As if something was being screwed into the leg. At night in bed. Hard pressure, gentle motion and doubling up relieve it.

Conium Maculatum

Common Hemlock (Poison Hemlock or Poison Parsley) is the poison reputedly used to kill Socrates. It is a common plant throughout the northern hemisphere. Because of its similarity to parsley it has sometimes been mistaken for it, with disastrous results. Every part of the plant is extremely poisonous. Paralysis starts at the feet and moves upward. The homoeopathic remedy is prepared from the whole plant gathered when it is in flower. The remedy is entirely harmless and not at all poisonous.

Causation: Blows, contusions.

Worse: Exertion, injury, lying down, night. Reading and using eyes. Celibacy.

Better: Hanging legs down, stooping, sitting down, dieting, in the sun.

Complaints: Epiphysitis of the calcaneum, sacroiliac injuries.

General Uses: Dizzy and sweating at night lying in bed after an accident or injury. Burning in eyes. Older athletes who recover slowly after injury may benefit from the remedy. Staggering when walking. Note the strange symptom that sitting with the legs hanging down relieves the condition.

Lower limbs: Shooting pains in the heel, with a feeling that there is a lump or stone under the heel and that the bone would push out. Legs feel paralysed.

Back: Conditions from injuries and overexertion that sprain the left side of the sacroiliac symphysis. Cramp-like, aching and compressive pain in the lower back is worse from bending backwards and twisting. It may feel as if there is a steel band around the sacrum. The pain prevents him turning in bed. It is worse from standing.

Mental/Emotional: Memory becomes weak, cannot concentrate or understand things said to him, unwilling to work. Depressed and timid. Worries about sexual abstinence and performance.

Cuprum Metallicum

The metal copper; the homoeopathic remedy is made by trituration.

Causation: Overexertion. Prolonged physical activity.

Worse: Exertion, movement, touch.

Better: Stretching the leg.

Complaints: Cramp.

Lower limbs: Violent cramps in the calves at night in bed, or after very strenuous prolonged physical activity and exertion. Knotted muscles. Stretching relieves. Intense pain.

Drosera

The plant *Drosera rotundifolia* is better known as the Sundew. It grows in wet marshy places in heaths, moorland and mountains. The plant is insectivorous, and was used to treat tuberculosis in early times.

Worse: After midnight, on lying down, laughing, singing.

Better: Pressure, open air.

Complaints: Cough.

General Uses: Deep, barking, hacking, tormenting cough. From tickling in the larynx. Pain in the chest. Holds his chest when coughing. Voice becomes deep and hoarse, The cough comes on as soon as his head touches the pillow. Typically the cough comes on after a cold, and is difficult to shift. The cough is so violent that it makes him vomit.

Elaps Corallinus

Elaps Corallinus is the Brazilian coral snake. The poison is extracted and used to make the remedy.

Worse: As storms approach, in a room, at night.

Better: Walking, rest.

Complaints: Nosebleed.

General Uses: If Arnica does not stop a nosebleed after two or three doses and the nose continues to bleed dark-coloured blood after a blow, with pain at the root of the nose. This remedy has the strange symptom that the nose bleeds in a room and stops when the person walks in the open air – but not when it is raining; hates rain.

Euphrasia

Eyebright is a pretty little white flower that grow in grasslands in northern Europe. It has been used as a remedy for eye complaints since ancient times.

Worse: Sunlight, wind, warmth, in room, rising from bed or chair.

Better: Open air, blinking and wiping eyes.

Complaints: Eye conditions. Hay fever. Inguinal pain.

General Uses: Eyes sore, water easily. Hay fever when the nose discharge is profuse but bland, and the hot watery discharge from the eyes makes them very sore and red. The opposite of Allium Cepa. Pain and soreness in an injured eye. This remedy will also relieve many eye symptoms such as discharge, soreness, conjunctivitis and pain especially when there is profuse, hot and acrid watering. Strain or sprain in the inguinal or rectal area. Stitching pain extends to the testes and rectum, when sitting. Stretching the legs aggravates it.

Ferrum Metallicum

Iron is the most common metal in earth's crust after aluminium and is one of the main constituents of the body.

Worse: Raising arms, sudden motion, lying down, at midnight.

Better: Gentle motion, leaning head on something.

Complaints: Mainly right shoulder. Rotator cuff injuries, tendinitis of shoulder, frozen shoulder.

Upper limbs: Frozen right shoulder, rotator cuff injury, tearing and stinging pain. Rheumatism of right shoulder. Insists on trying to lift the arm even though it is extremely painful to do so. Moving the arm is intensely painful. Lifts arm gingerly to relieve the pain. Cracking or crepitus in the joint, and the pain is worse at night when lying down.

Mental/Emotional: Jumpy. The least noise is unbearable. Much better when working or doing something. Anxiety and guilty feelings.

Gelsemium

Although the common name for this plant is Yellow Jasmine it should not be confused with the true jasmine. The plant is native to North America, where it is found in woodlands and on sea coasts. It belongs to the same family as Nux Vomica and Ignatia – the Loganiaceae – and is poisonous. The homoeopathic remedy is made from the fresh root. This is chopped and soaked in alcohol, and the resultant liquid succussed.

Causation: Hearing bad news. Anticipating an ordeal. Exhaustion.

Worse: Physical exertion, bad news, emotions.

Better: Sweating, urinating, mental tasks.

Complaints: Flu. Colds. Exhaustion. Overexertion. Stage fright, nerves, anticipation.

General Uses: Cold that takes several days to develop. Or a cold with the symptoms of 'flu comes on suddenly after exertion, exhaustion and stress. Sneezing, red face, heavy eyelids, cold limbs, shivering, aching in all joints, headache and drowsiness. Runny nose, headache, tired heavy aching eyes, aching bones and joints, sore throat when swallowing, face dusky red, overpowering need to lie down and rest.

Mental/Emotional: The person with flu symptoms who is very reluctant to give in and rest, and insists on trying to play or work. Stage fright and nerves. Shakes with fright, and dreads an ordeal. Almost paralysed with fear. Apathetic and indifferent to disguise his fright. Underneath he is very nervous. Very drowsy but cannot sleep from the excitement of anticipation. Loses appetite and thirst. Wobbly knees. Loss of skills from muscle tension. Cannot relax. This person reacts in a way that is opposite to the Argentum Nitricum personality – that person speeds up, whereas the Gelsemium person slows down.

Glonoine

Nitroglycerine is diluted with alcohol to make this remedy.

Worse: Heat, sun on head. Motion, jarring, shaking, travel.

Better: Shaded open air. Cold.

Complaint: Headache from too much sun. Heatstroke and exhaustion. Cannot bear to be in the sun. Eyes and face red. Worse from exposure to the sun or heat. Desires cold applications and shade.

Mental and Emotional: Confused, bewildered, weeps and shudders. Very irritable. Does not recognise people and places well know to her.

Graphites

This remedy is made from plumbago or black lead, the substance used to make the best pencils.

Causation: Overlifting.

Worse: Cold, warmth of bed, night.

Better: Walking in open air, drinking milk.

Complaints: Plantar fasciitis, spring ligament tear. Athlete's foot. Burning in soles and heels. Sore lips.

General Uses: Lips cracked and sore from cold, with gluey moisture.

Lower limbs: Shooting, tearing, burning pain in the soles. Folds between the toes become raw and moist and exude a smelly, gluey, honey-like moisture. Nails thick and ingrowing. Foul, acrid, excoriating sweat between toes. Plantar fasciitis with burning pain in bed.

Guaiacum

This remedy is prepared from the resin of the *Guaiacum* or 'Lignum Vitae' tree.

Worse: Heat, touch, motion, sitting.

Better: Cold applications.

Complaints: Torn meniscus.

Lower limbs: The knee remains flexed and there is tearing pain when trying to extend it. The least movement of the leg is very painful. Reluctant to move. Heat makes it worse, as does touch. Worse sitting, in the morning. Yawning and stretching. Growing pains in adolescents. Indolent.

Mental/Emotional: Obstinate with fixed ideas. Critical. Forgetful.

Hamamelis

The leaves and bark of Witch Hazel, the English name for *Hamamelis virginica*, are astringent and bitter. They were used by North American Indians as poultices for swellings and tumours. The lotion has become a household remedy for burns, scalds, insect bites and other inflammatory conditions. The shrub grows widely in North America. The bark is chopped and pounded, left to stand in alcohol for eight days, and then succussed and potentised.

Causation: Injuries.

Worse: Injuries, bruises, pressure, cold open air, touch, day time.

Complaints: Vaginal bruising, nosebleeds, varicose veins, piles.

General Uses: The vagina feels bruised and sore, tender, swollen and inflamed. There is bleeding, but the person seems surprisingly unconcerned and tranquil about it. The abdomen may also be sore and feel bruised. Does not want to move, and prefers to keep warm and stay indoors. Does not want ice or cold applications. Large sore, bruised feeling, bleeding piles that are worse in the open air, from sitting on hard cold surfaces. Nosebleed of thin dark blood in the morning.

Mental/Emotional: Surprisingly unconcerned and tranquil about condition. Feels unappreciated and wants respect.

Hecla Lava

This remedy is made from the volcanic ash of Mount Hecla in Iceland. Garth Wilkinson, a homoeopath travelling in Iceland, noticed that the local sheep developed huge exostoses on their jaws. Further clinical use of the remedy showed that it had the effect of reducing bony growths and diseases of bone. The remedy is made from fine volcanic ash, triturated and succussed.

Causation: Injuries to bone, muscles, tendons and ligaments.

Complaints: Calcaneum spur. Ectopic calcification and myositis ossificans.

Lower limbs: Any bony growths, and exostoses that are sensitive and painful to touch.

Hepar Sulphuris

The material from which this remedy is made was prepared by Hahnemann from oyster shell and flowers of sulphur. The resultant compound is also called calcium sulphide. The remedy is made by trituration.

Worse: Cold winds, draughts, night, touch, lying down.

Better: Heat, wrapping up warmly, especially the head.

Complaints: Cough. Cold. Sore throat. Wounds.

General Uses: Cough, barking and dry at night but loose and productive in the morning, from post nasal drip. Thick, yellow, sticky mucus. Colds, sneezing from uncovering, nasal catarrh drips down the back of the throat and is yellow and smelly. Bones of the nose feel sore and the sense of smell is lost. Sore throat, raw, splinter-like pain, from tonsils to the ear. It hurts to swallow, cough, even to turn the head and yawn. There is a sensation of a splinter or fish bone in the throat, and the tonsils are swollen with ulcers like white spots.

Mental/Emotional: Oversensitive to physical and mental hurt. Very irritable and violently angry. Very sensitive to draughts, will yell at anyone who leaves a door open, even in the next room.

Hydrastis

The North American plant known as Golden Seal produces an intense yellow dye. The remedy is made from the underground stem.

Worse: Breathing cold air, lying on back.

Better: Pressure. Sitting on hard edge.

Complaints: Groin strain and pain.

General Uses: Pain in the inguinal area that feels sprained when standing. The area feels sore, bruised and tender. The pain may be cutting or stabbing. It may extend into the testes. Whereas Euphrasia pain starts on the left, Hydrastis pain starts on the right and may extend up through the abdomen as far as the scapula. Pain is in the os pubis. Presses the painful area to relieve it. Sits on a hard edge. Lying on his back makes the pain worse, as does motion. He may therefore be reluctant to move. You should be aware that the female patient who needs Hydrastis could have a serious urogenital condition, and refer her accordingly.

Mental/Emotional: Wants to stay at home. Gloomy, taciturn, spiteful. Moaning – would rather be dead.

Hypericum

St John's Wort is found in hedgerows, woods and the edges of meadows, and is cultivated in gardens. Its yellow flowers exude a reddish/orange juice when crushed. The plant has been used since early times to treat deep wounds. The homoeopathic remedy is made from the crushed, whole, flowering plant. The juice is mixed with alcohol and succussed after standing for a week.

Causation: Bites, wounds, shock. Crushed and bruised toes and fingers.

Worse: Injury, jar, concussion, motion.

Better: Rubbing, lying on face, bending backwards.

Complaints: Wounds, injuries to coccyx and spine, nerve-rich parts, fingers and toes, bites, shooting pains. Genital injuries.

General Uses: Wounds, slow healing. Crushed, nerve rich parts, punctured, lacerated, with shooting pains. Violent and intolerable, shooting pain. Inflamed bites from animals and stings. Wounds after dentistry, surgery, splinters and accidents. Shooting pains in the genitals after a blow. The genitals are very painful and sore and very sensitive to touch, even of the clothing, and jarring. Movement is very painful. Blood in the urine as a result of injury.

Upper limbs: Bleeding under bruised nail causes unbearable and shooting pain into the hand and arm. Crushed, broken fingers. Bruised, painful nails. Violent, shooting piercing pain and soreness in nerve rich parts always respond to Hypericum. The fingers are very sensitive to touch and jarring. Much more painful than it appears. Better from rubbing. The athlete or dancer tends to rub it whenever possible.

Lower limbs: Pain unbearable and shooting into the foot and leg after bleeding under bruised nail. Broken toes.

Back: Injuries to the spine and coccyx. Pain is violent and intolerable. Shooting and cutting, aching and soreness in the coccyx and between the scapulae. The spine is painfully sensitive. Spasm in the muscles. Numbness following injury and concussion. Worse from movement. Cervical spine as much as any other part. The pain is violent and intolerable. There is stiffness aching and soreness. The neck is painfully sensitive. Muscle spasm.

Mental/Emotional: Fear and nervous depression following injuries. Sense of exhaltation and being high up before an accident. Fear of falling.

Ipecacuanha

This plant, as named by the Portuguese explorers of Central and South America, means 'Makes you sick'. The homoeopathic remedy is prepared from the root. It is dried and powdered, mixed with alcohol, and the liquor succussed.

Worse: At night. Warmth. Overeating. Motion. Abuse of drugs.

Better: Open air. Rest. Cold drinks.

Complaints: Nausea. Cough.

General: Nausea, persistent, constant, violent, with much empty belching, pale face, after eating, movement. The smell of food and tobacco smoke make him feel sick. Not better after vomiting. Persistent, incessant and violent cough. This is mostly a children's cough remedy, but worth remembering for adult use as well. Coughs until he vomits. Sudden fainting in hot weather.

Kali Carbonicum

Potassium carbonate is found in all plants, and was originally obtained from the ashes left after burning wood and vegetables. It has been used since earliest times in the manufacture of glass and is still used to make soap. Potassium is essential to the electrochemical processes in the heart as well as for reducing blood pressure. The homoeopathic remedy is prepared by trituration.

Causation: Overuse injuries, overstrain, catching cold, after over-heating.

Worse: Cold air, draughts, lying on painful side, sudden motion, 2 to 3 a.m.

Better: Warmth of bed, by day, open air, gentle motion.

Complaints: Foot pain, sciatica.

General: Exhaustion after a long season or tournament, when the person becomes very irritable and quarrelsome, catches colds easily, develops stomach problems through anxiety and weakness develops in arms and legs.

Lower limbs: Tearing pain in the sole caused by a sudden, unguarded movement. Very sensitive to touch. Does not like cold. Pain is worse in the middle of the night. Aching, sciatic, shooting pains extend to the tibia and ankle. Aching, shooting pains, very sensitive feet after a fracture.

Mental/Emotional: Anxious, bad-tempered and quarrelsome.

Lac Defloratum

This remedy is derived from skimmed milk.

Complaints: Constipation.

General: Constipation with ineffectual urging and great straining to pass a large hard stool. Pain radiates from below the sternum and across the abdomen at about the level of the umbilicus. Violent sick headache. Much stinking flatus that relieves the pain. Milk nauseates and aggravates the condition.

Mental/Emotional: Horror of being shut in, likes to leave doors open. Thinks and talks of death.

Lachesis

Poison from the Surukuku snake of South America. This snake poison remedy was discovered in 1828 and has been in use ever since. As a polychrest it has many uses for conditions generally affecting the left side of the body.

Worse: Sleep, morning, heat of sun, tight clothing

Better: Open air, cold drinks.

Complaints: Pain, left elbow, arm and hand. Headache. Sore throat. After sleeping.

General Uses: Headache on waking in the morning, after a sleep, and after exposure to heat and sun. Left sided sore throat that comes on in the morning and spreads rapidly into the ear and then to the other side.

Upper limbs: This remedy is particularly effective for the left elbow and hand when there is great weakness after overexertion. The condition comes on suddenly when the athlete or dancer wakes in the morning. Possible recurrence every two weeks. Pain in the elbow. The left arm is numb and weak, and tingling in the hand. General weakness. Movement makes it worse.

Lower limbs: Sciatica in the left leg on waking. Makes it impossible to move it.

Mental/Emotional: Talks a lot about many subjects. The most talkative person you know. Jealous, suspicious, nervous and excitable. Wakes miserable. Fears going to sleep. May be very religious.

Ledum

Wild Rosemary, *Ledum palustre*, grows in marshes and bogs in Europe and America. It has a strong, resinous smell, and is reputed to keep away lice and prevent flour from getting mouldy. It has been used as a substitute for hops in beer making, but the resultant unpleasant drunkenness with headache and dizziness stopped that practice. The remedy is produced from the small twigs and leaves, which are dried and powdered, mixed with alcohol and the liquor succussed.

Causation: Puncture wounds, bites, stings, wounds, bruises.

Worse: Warmth, motion of injured joint, night.

Better: Cold bathing, rest.

Complaints: Sesamoiditis. Osteochondritis. Sore feet. Ankle sprain. Torn meniscus. Black eye. Puncture and lacerated wounds. Bites and stings.

General Uses: For bloodshot and bruised eyes, with bruising and discoloration, the top eyelid droops over the eye (ptosis). Black eye, following Arnica, to help the bruising come out. After bites and stings, to prevent infection. Ledum will prevent infection in puncture and lacerated wounds.

Lower limbs: Sesamoiditis. Pain is felt behind the toes and movement makes the pain worse, Swelling and tenderness. Cold applications ease the pain and warmth makes it worse. Soles so sore that the person avoids stepping on them. Tenderness and loose swelling in the pad behind the big toe or hallux. Pain is worse, and the back of the foot itches at night. Feet very stiff on first rising in the morning. A strange symptom for Ledum is that the soles are most painful on walking upstairs. Ankles which sprain easily and frequently. Suspected osteoarthritis. Joints painful, and oedematous. Tearing pains, weakness and numbness. Although the foot and ankle may be cold, the person is worse from warmth. Moving the joint is painful. Cold bathing ameliorates. Torn meniscus with bruising and swelling.

Lycopodium

Alpine club moss grows freely on heaths and mountains throughout northern Europe. The spores of the moss are used to make the remedy. They are potentised by trituration.

Worse: Between 4 p.m. and 8 p.m., and on waking. Warmth, cold food, vegetables.

Better: Warm drinks and food.

Complaints: Torn meniscus. Nerves. Indigestion and stomach upsets.

General: Very bloated with wind, with burning, acid pain in stomach. Hungry, but full after a few mouthfuls. Bread, soup, pasta, cold foods disagree. Nervous indigestion before a match or performance and eats only little.

Lower limbs: Tearing pain prevents extension of a locked knee. The knee gives way suddenly. Heat treatment relieves the pain, but he dislikes a warm room. Pressure hurts. Injuries to the right knee. Right-sided sciatica.

Mental/Emotional: Loses self-confidence when faced with doing something new, or performing in a new environment. Angry, anxious and hurried. Very nervous before playing or performing, but overcomes the nerves as the game or performance begins. Loves the challenge of new places, but anxiety and anger affect performance adversely. Lacks courage in rehabilitation after injury.

Magnesia Carbonica

Magnesium carbonate.

Worse: Rest, every other day, night, touch, change of weather.

Better: Walking about, motion, open air.

Complaints: Baker's cyst.

Lower limbs: This is a specific remedy for Baker's cyst when there is swelling in the popliteal, and especially for the left knee. Cannot put left foot to the ground. But likes to walk about in the open air because he feels better. The pain seems to be worse every other day, and is better from motion.

Mental/Emotional: Anxious, sad, in bed. Insomnia after 3 a.m.

Magnesia Phosphorica

Magnesium phosphate is found in many tissues in the body and has an affinity for nervous and muscular tissue. The homoeopathic remedy and the tissue salt has the reputation for relieving muscle spasms, and conditions attributable to them.

Worse: Cold air, draughts, cold water, night.

Better: Warmth, hot bathing, pressure, rubbing, doubling up.

Complaints: Prolapsed intervertebral disc. Lower back pain. Cramps.

Lower limbs: Cramps from prolonged exertion.

Back: Cramps, convulsions and neuralgic spasmodic pains come on suddenly. Worse by touch. Stiffness and cramps in the back at night. Every two weeks, every six months or similarly. An athlete or dancer reaches the end of a long, exhausting tournament or season and, after relaxing, suddenly develops a prolapsed disc.

Mental/Emotional: Always talking about his injuries or pains.

Mercurius Solubilis

Mercury was almost the only orthodox medical treatment available for several diseases, including syphilis and gonorrhoea, in the 19th century. Its extreme toxicity led Hahnemann to try to discover an alternative even before he had discovered his system of homoeopathic medicine. He invented a compound of mercury with ammonium nitrate, which was non-corrosive and soluble. He later proved it as a homoeopathic remedy, and it has become one of our polychrests.

There are two commonly used homoeopathic remedies called Mercurius. These are Merc. Solubilis and Merc. Corrosivus. Be careful when you order or purchase either so that you get the one you want.

Worse: Sweating, being hot, night, draughts, getting the feet wet.

Better: Rest.

Complaints: Mouth ulcers. Sore throat. Toothache.

General Uses: Painful ulcers in the cheeks and gums and behind the lips, with much salivation and really offensive bad breath. Raw, burning, sore throat. Difficult, painful swallowing with pain into the ears. Breath so bad you can smell it from six feet away. Indented tongue, much saliva. Sweetish metallic taste in mouth. Toothache, pain worse at night in bed, perhaps from an abscess, aggravated by draughts and cold air, tooth feels bruised, cheek swollen, pain spreads to ears, face and head, much saliva, and very bad breath.

Mental/Emotional: Speaks hurriedly. Restless, forgetful, slows down and becomes lethargic when sick, but feels hurried and panicky inside.

Natrum Arsenicum

Sodium Arsenicum.

Complaints: Nausea from a blow to the genitals. Must be referred for medical treatment immediately.

Natrum Muriaticum

Despite being one of the most widely distributed substances in the world, common salt – sodium chloride – is one of the most surprising and effective homoeopathic remedies. Its range of action includes almost every known clinical condition. Its use in the sports injury field depends on the totality of the person's symptoms. If you suspect a person needs a deep-acting constitutional remedy such as this, it is important that he or she should be referred for qualified homoeopathic evaluation.

Causation: Old disappointments, grief, old grudges.

Worse: Sympathy and consolation, 9 to 11 a.m., alternate days, heat, exertion.

Better: Open air, being alone.

Complaints: Headache. Cold sores. Colds. Cracked lip. Osgood-Schlatter disease. Bursitis. Prolapsed disc. Groin pain.

General Uses: Headache from excitement, comes on at 11 a.m. Cold sores on the lips and around the mouth from tiredness, stress, anxiety and exposure to sun. Persistent painful cracks in the middle of the lower lip. Colds, the nose runs 'like a tap', gushing hot watery discharge and early morning sneezing. Take one Natrum Muriaticum 30c as soon as the symptoms appear.

Paroxysmal, neuralgic groin pain, worse when stretching, coughing, lying, rising and walking. The groin feels sprained, and the pain radiates along the spermatic chord. Tension in the inguinal ring.

Upper limbs: Numbness and tingling in the fingers with trembling of the hands when writing or performing delicate tasks. Cracks in the finger tips.

Lower limbs: Osgood-Schlatter disease, wrenching pain in knee when walking or standing. Restlessness and jerking of legs, cracking in knees during movement. Bursitis, 'housemaid's knee'. Any pressure on the knee is painful. Trembling, tingling and numbness. The condition comes on periodically, every other day, every day at a certain time, 9 to 11 a.m., or every week.

Back: Almost the opposite of Rhus Tox. – Natrum Mur. cannot straighten the back but can stoop easily. Paralysis in the lumbar region with painful stiffness. Spine very sensitive. Tearing pains that pulsate across sacroiliac and into hips. Tension and pulling in the back. Bruised backache worse early in the morning and again between 9 and 11 a.m. Hurts to cough, and is better when lying on back on something hard.

Mental/Emotional: A detached sort of person who does not get involved with other people's problems. 'Reserved' is a good description. A predominantly female remedy, but men may present the

247

symptoms. Angry. Detests fuss or consolation. Remembers old disappointments and grudges, and punishes people by being injured. Suppresses grief, but suffers from it. Worries about security and dreams of being robbed or losing things.

Natrum Sulphuricum

Glauber's Salt is used in manufacturing processes for paper, board, glass, dyeing and tanning. The remedy is made by trituration.

Causation: Following head injuries.

Worse: Night, early morning at 4 to 5 a.m., damp weather, lifting, touch, pressure.

Better: Lying on back, open air.

Complaints: Head injuries.

General Uses: Long-lasting and persistent symptoms following a head injury. If Arnica has been given and does not seem to work. Dizziness with nausea and vomiting. Confusion and irritability that was not present before the injury. Sensitive to noise and music. Crushing, bursting and nauseating, throbbing and violent headache. Very drowsy. Brain feels loose. Feels head is in a vice. Headache is better lying in a dark room.

Mental/Emotional: Depressed, even suicidal, but considers his family too much to commit suicide. Worse from concentration on mental work.

Nitric Acid

The homoeopathic remedy is made from nitric acid by evaporation and succussion.

Worse: Touch, jarring, cold air, night, motion.

Better: Steady pressure, mild weather.

Complaints: Anterior knee pain. Piles.

General Uses: Piles. Burning, worse after stool, like a splinter in the anus with easy bleeding, agony when walking. Itching, worse from touch, and warmth of bed.

Lower limbs: Splinter-like pain in the patella that makes walking difficult, and extends to the tibia. Worse from cold, touch and jarring.

Mental/Emotional: Violent anger. A very nasty temperament. Taciturn and quarrelsome. Drives himself to train and perform better. Cannot forgive anyone who has upset him. Very sensitive to noise and pain.

Nux Vomica

The Nux Vomica or Poison Nut tree grows throughout Asia. Its name means 'vomiting nut', and as such it had some limited use as an emetic to treat various diseases in the 19th century.

The homoeopathic remedy has wide uses. Like many of our great polychrests, if the person's symptoms fit those of the remedy it will cure their illness, whether it was caused by a sports injury or anything else. I have used it for hangovers, hips, indigestion, knees, elbows and backs in many cases, and have cured post-traumatic conditions with it.

The seeds are ground up with lactose sugar and triturated.

Causation: Anger, coffee, alcohol, injury, foreign food and travel.

Worse: Early morning, 3 a.m., open air, cold, coffee, over-eating and drinking.

Better: Vomiting, resting. Warm drinks.

Complaints: Hangover. Hay fever. Constipation. Headaches. Indigestion and stomach upsets. Insomnia. Nausea.

General Uses: Head feels heavy, with pressing, sore, tearing, stupefying, bruised pain. Biliousness, nausea and dizziness. Headache wakes him at 3 a.m., after drinking too much alcohol or eating too much rich food. Eyes feel sore. Hay fever with sneezing, runny nose during the day that blocks up at night, better in the open air, worse in the morning. Very irritable, headache, sore throat and a very runny nose.

Constipation. Uneasy feeling in bowels with urging to defecate, but without result. Bowels inactive. Would feel better if only he could go. Tenderness and cutting pain in the lower abdomen. Irritable when constipated. Constipation with other stomach upsets. Indigestion, heartburn and aversion to food.

Indigestion. Food lies like a stone in the stomach. After eating rich food and drinking alcohol, coffee and late nights. Acid rising into the throat. Many foods disagree. One of the first remedies to think of for indigestion.

Nausea. Constant after eating and drinking too much, in the morning, in bed, after breakfast, at the thought or smell of food. Feels altogether better after vomiting.

Insomnia. Cannot sleep from rush of ideas, or wakes very early, about 3 a.m., and cannot get to sleep again.

Lower limbs: Knees dry and cracking when walking.

Back: So sore he cannot turn in bed without sitting up.

Mental/Emotional: Workaholic. Stimulated by work and success. Very irritable, angry and impatient. An aggressive go-getter at work, and high achiever at play. Excited and stimulated by even small successes at sport. Hates it when other people ask him questions. Enjoys a drink and good food too much. Self-indulgent. Impulsive, critical, fussy and demanding; ignores the rules. Treats injury as a sign of courage.

Opium

The white poppy is native to Asia Minor, and is cultivated in Asia and South America for its opium. This is extracted from the poppy heads before they ripen. It was used as a sedative and pain reliever in ancient times. Codeine and morphine are both derived from it. The homoeopathic remedy is prepared by dissolving opium in alcohol and succussing. None of the original opium remains in the remedy.

Worse: Excitement, emotions, fear, fright.

Better: Cold, constant walking.

Complaints: Constipation. Head injury.

General Uses: Constipation. Absolutely no desire for stool and no urging. In hot weather. Throbbing in the abdomen and a feeling as if the anus were closed. Bowels feel completely obstructed and paralysed. Cannot pass flatus although his abdomen feels distended and hard. As if he as a weight inside.

Head injury when there has been complete loss of consciousness. He fears a repetition of the injury. Lightheaded. Eyes glassy and staring, pupils dilated or contracted or insensible to light. He falls into a heavy, coma like sleep, and snores loudly.

Mental/Emotional: This person is placid, dull, sluggish and lacks will-power when constipated, and talkative, happy and lively when he is well.

He becomes very placid, apart from his fear, and says that there is nothing wrong with him (like Arnica). He is dreamy yet talkative, lacks willpower, or is nervous and irritable. Not as fearful of touch as Arnica.

Paeonia

The remedy is made from the root of the peony flower.

Worse: Touch, pressure, night, walking.

Complaint: Haemorrhoids. Anal fissure.

General Uses: Very painful piles that itch. Excruciating pain in anus makes the person walk about at night. Debilitating piles with anal fissure and ulcers.

Phosphoric Acid

This remedy is made from a dilute solution of phosphoric acid.

Worse: Draughts, cold, emotion, music.

Better: Short sleep.

Complaint: Homesickness.

Mental/Emotional: Homesickness. Quiet, indifferent, apathetic, and brooding. Emotional, disinterested and tired. Aversion to talking. Weeps with homesickness. Weakness and lethargy. Sleepy during the day but sleeps badly at night. Reluctant to get going and start anything.

Phosphorus

The element phosphorus is the favourite of most chemistry teachers. If it is taken from the water or alcohol in which it is normally kept it bursts into a white flame spontaneously. This delights classes of children. It also glows in the dark. In the form of phosphates it is found throughout nature. The homoeopathic remedy is made by trituration, and is another of our great polychrests with a huge range of action.

Causation: Sprains. Lifting. Wounds. Exertion.

Worse: Lying on painful side, on left side, cold, emotional upset.

Better: Sleep, eating, cold.

Complaints: Tendinitis of shoulder. Shin splints. Nosebleed. Bleeding wounds. Cough. Phosphorus may often be appropriate for young dancers with very flexible joints.

General Uses: If Arnica does not stop the bleeding from any wound, which is profuse, bright red and restarts easily. Chronic and persistent epistaxis (nosebleed) of bright red blood, perhaps with clots. Brought on by blowing the nose, exertion, sweating, rubbing the nose. Especially for young people who seem to have grown too fast. Bleeding after tooth extraction.

Dry hard cough with tickling behind the sternum, wakes the person at night. Has to sit up to cough. Cough on going from a warm room out into the cold air. Exhausting cough. Cold drinks ease it, but they are vomited a short time later. Pain in the abdomen, with wheezing, burning in the air passages and trembling.

Upper limbs: Tearing pain in the left shoulder that is worse at night. Weakness in the affected arm on exertion, sometimes with trembling. From overlifting and overuse generally. Gradual onset. The joint is stiff without pain. Sleeping on the left side makes it worse. Worse in the morning and evening, and when tired. Likes massage. The shoulder condition comes and goes with the weather.

Lower limbs: Inflammation of the periosteum with tearing pain in the tibia. after exhaustion. Worse from any and every exertion. Tottery, stumbles easily. Legs heavy. Feet feel stuck to the floor.

Mental/Emotional: A very affectionate and sensitive person who cares much for others, she hates to be alone. Very excitable and impressionable. Fears thunderstorms. Clairvoyant. Demands sympathy.

Picric Acid

This acid was discovered by Hahnemann in 1788 when he observed the action of nitric acid on carbolic acid. The homoeopathic remedy is made by trituration of the yellow crystals.

Causation: Overexertion. Prolonged activity. Fatigue.

Worse: Mental and physical exertion. Fatigue. Shock.

Better: Rest.

Complaint: Exhaustion.

General Uses: Totally exhausted in body and mind. Weak, tired and heavy feeling. Aching, tired limbs. Wants only to rest. Sleepless from exhaustion, sleeps only restlessly, and feels 'too tired to sleep'

Mental/Emotional: Lacks will power. Deeply fears failure. Mental strain and anxiety. Sits still and lifeless. No interest in anything.

Piper Methysticum

The root of this Polynesian plant provides the stimulant kava. Tea made from it is drunk or the root is chewed before religious rites or important business undertakings. The remedy is made from a tincture of the root. It is reported that one dose of this remedy enables one to exercise without fatigue. More than two doses will, however, produce torpor and intense tiredness. The remedy was first used in very low potency, 1x, but potencies of 6c and higher are reported to have the same effect.

Causation: Exhaustion.

Better: Moving in the open air. Thinking about something else.

Worse: Before meals.

Complaint: Exhaustion, yet needs to continue.

General Uses: Weakness with trembling. Unable to stand. Stimulation to exertion without fatigue. Vertigo, swimming sensation and faintness. Sleeplessness at night, yet sleepy by day.

Mental/Emotional: Exhaltation of mind. All mental faculties sharpened, is capable of working for long periods without fatigue. Restless. Lazy and drowsy. Excited and highly-strung. Cheerful. Enjoys dancing and entertainment. Eats hurriedly. Suddenly becomes bored and lifeless. Solitary, dull and sleepy.

Plumbum Metallicum

Many of the symptoms for lead have been derived from poisonings among workers such as painters and plumbers. For many years the metal was considered inert and of little use as an orthodox medicine. It has been used by homoeopaths since the early days. The remedy is made by trituration.

Worse: Exertion in the open air in clear weather. Touch.

Better: Hard pressure, rubbing, stretching.

Complaints: Tenosynovitis of wrist and forearm.

General Uses: Violent cramps and contractions after exertion, with lightning-like pains.

Upper limbs: Painful weakness of the wrist and hand. The wrist feels paralysed and may be dropped. Difficulty in grasping objects. The symptoms appear very slowly and insidiously. Sensation of a string pulling the wrist into extension or flexion. Violent contraction of the fingers. Weakness and emaciation of the wrist after injury.

Mental/Emotional: A taciturn sort of person who is not keen on company. Slow thinking, he becomes even slower after exertion. Avoids being touched because it hurts. Avoids exertion, but likes a hard massage.

Podophyllum

The May Apple is a plant native to America. It was used by Native North Americans to cure intestinal worms and as a drastic laxative or purgative. Settlers used it to 'purge' the system. The homoeopathic remedy is made from the pulp of the root, gathered before the fruit is ripe. The pulp is strained with alcohol and succussed.

Worse: Immediately after drinking contaminated water. After eating, Hot weather. At 4 a.m. At night.

Better: Lying on abdomen.

Complaints: Diarrhoea.

General Uses: Much terrible gurgling and rumbling in abdomen, with dull ache or cramping pains. Then profuse painless putrid stools gush out, accompanied by loud wind. Feels totally drained, faint and weak. The rectum soon fills up again and they have to 'go' again. Frequent diarrhoea. Stool shoots out involuntarily instead of wind.

Mental/Emotional: Thinks he is going to die or is very seriously ill. Fidgety and restless. Cannot sit still. Restless, moaning.

Pulsatilla

This remedy is made from the Pasque Flower, or Wind Flower, *Pulsatilla nigricans*. It grows in meadows in northern Europe, and was used in country districts to treat ulcers and inflammations of the eye. The homoeopathic remedy is made from the whole plant, gathered when in flower.

Causation: Chill. Rich food. Fats.

Worse: Warm, stuffy rooms. Warm weather. Sitting in the sun. Lying down. Some time after eating. Rich, fatty food. Tobacco smoke.

Better: Gentle walking in fresh, open air. Cold. Standing upright. Pressure, rubbing.

Complaints: Headache. Indigestion. Insomnia. Nausea. Heel pain. Chronic knee swelling. Menstrual problems.

General Uses: The remedy is most often needed by slim, young, fair-haired people, but not exclusively so. Headache, pulsating, one sided, in a stuffy warm room, better in the open air. Delayed or absent periods. As a polychrest it will help any condition if the mental and general symptoms and modalities fit.

Indigestion. From fats, rich foods, toast, onions, tobacco smoke, tea, ice cream, cakes, warm food and drink. Comes on long after eating. Differentiate from Nux Vomica by the personality.

Insomnia. Thoughts go round and round in the head preventing sleep. Frequent waking; restless, anxious dreams. Overactive mind.

Nausea from rich fatty food, tobacco, with sensation of heavy weight in the stomach, some time after eating, with sour risings, dry mouth but no thirst.

Lower limbs: The young athlete or dancer experiences pain down the sides of the heel when beginning to walk, and in the evening. Continued swelling of the knee comes and goes without a pattern. The swelling may be hot and painful, or cold and white. The pain may wander to other limbs or places. Disinclined to stand for long.

Mental/Emotional: Mild-mannered, timid, tearful, easy-going, and enjoys sympathy. Very emotional, and change moods easily. Enjoys the sympathy from being injured. Pulsatilla is often required as a constitutional remedy for fair-haired young people who may be a bit weepy. Likely to forget the pain as soon as the mind is taken by another interest. Moody, sensitive, easily moved to tears. Needs company. Fears losing friends.

Rescue Remedy

Bach Rescue Remedy is included in this book although it is not a homoeopathic remedy. It is made from five flowering plants by suffusing them in water for some time, straining the liquid and adding two drops to a liquid ounce of alcohol and water.

I have used it in emergencies as a first contact remedy after accidents or trauma to relieve anxiety and panic with fainting, trembling and failing of physical capacity. I would always include it in my first aid kit.

Because it is not diluted to the same extent as a homoeopathic remedy care should be taken with its administration, as it may contain substances unacceptable for drug control.

Causation: Falls, blows, trauma, anxiety.

Complaints: Fainting, shivering, fright, pain, restlessness, insomnia, travel.

General Uses: For shock after injury or trauma, the person is anxious, chilled, and shivering. It can relieve pain in general. Excellent for insomnia from restlessness, fright and anxiety.

Mental/Emotional: Restlessness, anxiety and insomnia.

Rhododendron

The yellow Siberian Rhododendron is used for this remedy. The leaves are gathered when the seed pods have formed, and a tincture made from them.

Causation: Sprains. Storms.

Worse: Before storms. Rough windy weather. Cold, damp nights. Getting wet. Rest.

Better: After storm begins. First motion. Hot sunshine.

Complaints: Groin injuries. Heel pain. Stress fractures. Tenosynovitis of wrist and forearm. Arthritis and rheumatism. Recovery from sprains and fractures.

General Uses: When the testes are swollen, painful, feel crushed, and are drawn up after injury. The scrotum may be inflamed. There is a drawing pain from the spermatic cord into the abdomen and thighs. Injury to the glans penis when it feels crushed. The pain may be tearing, and he feels paralysed.

Upper limbs: Wrist bruised and sprained. The pain is tearing, and there is a sensation of boring. Stiffness, paralysis and weakness in the wrist and hand. The pain is worse at night and at rest. Unlike Rhus Tox., which is painful on first movement, Rhododendron is better as soon as movement begins.

Lower limbs: Bruised, drawing and tearing pain in the heel. The feet feel cold, even in a warm room and in bed. Weakness after even slight exertion. Heat reduces the discomfort. Drawing, tearing pain in tibia. Feels as if he has a weight on his foot. Feet are cold. Better from heat, and better immediately he starts moving. (Rhus Tox. is better after the first few movements.) Slight exertion makes him exhausted and weak.

Back: Pains in sacrum when sitting.

Mental/Emotional: Easily affected by alcohol. Forgets what he is talking about. Fear of thunder.

Rhus Toxicodendron

The Poison Ivy is native to North America, growing in woods, meadows and along fences. It was introduced to Europe in 1640 and has been used as a homoeopathic medicine since 1798. Its properties were discovered when a French doctor noticed that after an accidental poisoning with the plant a patient was cured of a longstanding eczematic condition.

It is a major remedy for conditions which are worse for first movement and better for continued movement, for those that are worse on cold, wet nights, and when the person is resting. It has been the subject of conventional medical testing as a 'catch all' cure for arthritis. Unfortunately, all the tests have disregarded the basic principle of homoeopathy – that is to say, a remedy is most effective when selected according to the totality of the patient's symptoms.

The remedy is prepared from fresh leaves gathered at night when the poison is most active. They are chopped and pounded to a pulp, left standing in alcohol, strained and succussed. It can, of course, be prescribed successfully for local conditions if the symptoms fit those of the remedy.

Causation: Cold. Becoming chilled after exertion. Overexertion, unaccustomed long-term exertion, repetitive strain, overuse injuries. Overlifting.

Worse: Rest, beginning movement. Exposure to wet cold weather, cold or draught when hot and sweaty. After midnight. Before storms. Overexertion. Lying on the injured side.

Better: Continued movement. Changing position. Heat, hot bathing. Stretching. Warm dry weather.

Complaints: Adhesions. Ankle sprains, tears and fractures. Arthritis. Arthritic complaints and pains. Bony growths and exostoses. Foot pain.

Heel pain. Inflammation of joints, tendons and ligaments with rheumatic pains. Injuries to genitals. Osgood-Schlatter disease. Osteoarthritis. Plantar fasciitis or tear. Rheumatoid arthritis. Soreness and bruising. Stiffness on first moving. Stiffness after unaccustomed and strenuous exertion. Sprains and strains. Sensation of joint being dislocated. Shin splints.

General Uses: Sprains, strains, stiffness from unaccustomed exertion or activity. Pains after traumatic injury, overexertion and overlifting. Long-term exertion, overuse or misuse. It has a special affinity with bony outgrowths, and has been known to reduce them if the patient manifests other Rhus Tox. symptoms. Stitching, burning, aching, tearing, shooting pains. Inflammation and swelling in testes. Scrotum thick, swollen and oedematous.

Upper limbs: During recovery from injury, especially if first movement is painful and continued movement relieves the pain. Tearing and burning sensation in the shoulder, worse when resting, and in bed. The right arm is weak and feels rheumatic. Tenosynovitis of the elbow. The athlete or dancer moves the arm constantly. Paralysing and nauseating pain in either elbow. Centred in the humeral epicondyle. The elbow is hot, swollen and painful. Arm feels shaky. Tenosynovitis of the wrist and forearm.

Lower limbs: Sore and painful feet, especially brought on by unusual and excessive exertion. Feet hot and painful, stiff and paralysed. Stitching, burning or aching in the sole of the foot. Pain as if 'stepping on a stone'. Worse in the morning, on waking and on rising, after sitting.

Ankle hot, painful and swollen, worse in the evening. Tearing, shooting or stitching, worse at night and at rest. First movement painful but continued movement relieves the pain. Cannot rest, gets up and walks around at night. Ankle swells after sitting or lying, and in the evening. Better after a hot bath.

Soreness in tibia at night and in bed. The leg feels sore and bruised, and as if the flesh was torn from the bone. Inflammation and swelling. Has to keep moving the leg because it feels better then. Restless.

All knee conditions worse on first movement, rising from a seat or in the morning, but better with continuous movement. Sore pain and stiffness at night. Worse when lain on. After strenuous activity.

Hamstring tears when the athlete has warmed up well, then cooled down, and then gone into a violent surge of effort such as a sprint start.

Back: Lower back pain. Many typical physical symptoms of lower back pain fit Rhus Tox. almost exactly, and I would expect it to eliminate pain in those cases. The back is stiff with painful tension when first moving. It is better from stretching, bending backwards and walking about, and also from lying on a hard surface. Pain following exertion, lifting. Rest, sitting and lying aggravate the pain, and movement ameliorates it. Heat and hot bathing ameliorate. Contractive backache. The back feels as if it would break on first moving. Hard pressure eases it. At rest and at night the pain radiates down the thigh. Typically the person wakes early from the pain, cannot find a comfortable position in bed, is restless and cannot sleep. The pain extends down the sciatic nerve and makes him even more restless. He has to get up early and walk around. Eventually he becomes exhausted mentally and physically, depressed, anxious and irritable.

Mental/Emotional: Very restless, cannot sit still or rest in any one position. Anxiety, sadness, profound despondency, with thoughts of suicide. Discouraged, discontented and irritable. Concentration difficult. All worse after midnight. Likes to be alone and believes he has been ostracised by his friends. Disturbed nights with dreams of great exertion. Cannot lie in bed and gets up to pace about restlessly. Mentally exhausted from lack of sleep.

Warning: It may be tempting to take a remedy such as Rhus Tox. frequently over a long period of time. There is a danger of developing other and deeper symptoms from the long-term repetition of any remedy which has been found to be effective in the short term.

Rumex Crispus

The common dock grows almost everywhere in hedgerows, meadows and untended gardens. Traditionally it cures nettle rash. It is also a traditional country remedy for constipation, cancer, diphtheria and obstinate skin diseases. The homoeopathic remedy is made from the root, which is chopped, pounded and the juice strained from the pulp.

Worse: Breathing cold air, becoming cold, lying down.

Better: Wrapping up.

Complaints: Cough.

General Uses: Dry, hacking cough in the morning. Extremely sensitive to cold air causing tickling in the throat pit and a continuous cough.

Going from a warm room to a cold one, or vice versa. (Phosphorus is worse on going from warm to cold.) Breathing, lying down, night, talking and uncovering all make the cough worse. Pain under the sternum. He may cover his mouth with his hands, even when he is not coughing.

Mental/Emotional: Keeps a blanket or towel over his head and face to prevent breathing the cold air. Very restless.

Ruta Graveolens

This remedy is made from rue, a native of southern Europe that grows wild almost anywhere on dry soil. Its common names include Herb of Grace. The name rue derives from the Greek 'reuo', meaning 'to set free', because the herb was efficacious in treating so many diseases. Shakespeare mentions it in Richard III: 'I'll set a bank of rue, sour herb of grace.' Rue water was sprinkled in houses to keep away fleas. The homoeopathic remedy is made from the fresh herb, chopped, pounded and the juice expressed. It is allowed to stand in alcohol and succussed.

Ruta may be considered a specific remedy for injuries to fibrous tissue, ligaments, tendons and cartilage, and for the main joints such as ankles, wrists, knees, shoulders and hips.

Causation: Overexertion, injury, sprains, overuse.

Worse from: Cold, damp or wet weather, lying on the injured limb, sitting, overexertion, ascending or descending steps, lying, sitting.

Better from: Warmth, rubbing, gentle motion, rest if he can find a comfortable position, but too much rest makes him worse. Lying on back.

Complaints: Strained and damaged ligaments, tendons and cartilage. Inflammation of tendons and ligaments. Deep bruising of the periosteum. Bruised, sore, aching joints and connective tissue. Pain deep in the long bones. Foot pain, heel pain, plantar fasciitis, Achilles tendon tears and strains, ankle sprain, fracture and dislocation. Shin splints, tibia pain, muscle tears. Hamstring tears. Collateral and meniscus tears. Rotator cuff tears and strains.

General Uses: Use Ruta to aid recovery after any injury involving ligaments, tendons or cartilage, whether from trauma or overuse. It is very useful after prolonged strenuous exertion, when the effects show in tendons and ligaments. Sleeps badly with frequent waking, yawning. Restlessness, has to move to get comfortable. Lameness, weakness, parts lain on become sore. Stiffness in tendons better after movement.

Upper limbs: Wrenching pain in shoulder, especially when arms hang down. Acute rotator cuff tears. Fibrosis and thickening of the tendon. Tendinitis in the rotator cuff and shoulder. Injuries to the sterno-clavicular joint and strains to the acromioclavicular and coraco-clavicular ligaments. Will reduce painful swelling over the acromio-clavicular joint and reduce pain on scapulothoracic movement. Aids repair of the ligaments after dislocation. Helps to prevent recurrent dislocation of glenohumeral joint. Dull pain in elbow and feeling of contusion. Tennis elbow. Epicondylitis and tenosynovitis in the elbow. Tears and sprains to elbow ligaments. Bones and joints feel as if they have been beaten. Pain in wrist when lifting weight, wrist feels sprained. Instability of wrist after damage to ligaments.

Lower limbs: Spring ligament strains. Legs feel weak and unsteady, especially ascending or descending stairs. Weakness in hip and thigh when rising from a seat. Feeling of contraction in tendons of knee. Aching in hip, knee and/or ankle. Lameness in the ankle after injury, sprain or dislocation. Ankles swollen, rheumatic pain in ankles. Hamstrings feel short. Pain in hip after unaccustomed stretching, especially when arthritic conditions are suspected. Laxity or rupture of the cruciate ligaments causing weakness and unsteadiness. Knee gives way on ascending and descending steps. Infrapatellar tendinitis, sprained medial and lateral ligaments. Suspected meniscus tears. Shin splints and peroneus tertius tendinitis. Acute ankle sprains, peritendinitis and tendinitis of Achilles tendon.

Back: Drawing pain in neck and between scapulae. Shooting pain in lumbar region when walking, bending and sitting, or only when sitting. Lumbar region feels bruised. Backache, better from pressure and when lying on the back. Pain in coccyx after a fall.

Mental/Emotional: Depressed about recovery, dissatisfied with himself and others about his injury, and after prolonged exertion. Despair of recovery, says 'This is probably the end of my playing days.' Anxious and guilty about being injured. Painful weariness. Unwilling to do rehabilitative exercises.

Sabadilla

Derived from a member of the Veratrum family of plants.

Worse: Smell of flowers. Even from thought of flowers. Smell of garlic.

Better: Open air.

Complaints: Hay fever.

General Uses: Persistent violent sneezing with itching and tickling in the nose. The symptoms come on regularly at set periods, every two or four weeks, or at the same time every year. Watery discharge. Eyelids red and burning. Eyes watering. Dizziness, must put head on table to relieve it. One-sided headache.

Mental/Emotional: Tends to be miserable with the condition.

Sanguinaria Canadensis

Blood Root is a native North American plant. Dye from the root was used by North American Indians to colour their faces and bodies, and later by dyers to colour cloth. The homoeopathic remedy is made from the juice extracted from the chopped and pounded root.

Worse: Raising arms, touch, as the sun climbs, weekly.

Better: Sleep.

Complaints: Rotator cuff and tendon tears.

Upper limbs: Cutting or stabbing pain felt in the right deltoid, worse on raising the arm. A feeling of rheumatism in the right shoulder. The shoulder pain is much worse at night, and seems to be in the surface bones, the acromion, and the greater tuberosity. Neuralgic pain which is relieved by touching the part. The pain may also be relieved by swinging the arm back and fore. The shoulder feels burning hot.

Mental/Emotional: Better after a good sleep, but may be morose. Grumbles about things. Dreamy. Optimistic of recovery.

Sanicula

This remedy is potentised spring water from Lake Sanicula, Ottawa, Illinois.

Worse: Raising arms, putting them behind back.

Better: Warmth.

Complaints: Rotator cuff tears and strains.

Upper limbs: This remedy is indicated specifically when the pain is worse from putting the hands behind the back and when raising the arms. The condition originates with strain and is worse from motion.

Mental/Emotional: Headstrong, obstinate and irritable, and does not want to be touched. Fears the dark.

Sepia

Hahnemann noticed that a sickly artist friend frequently licked his paintbrush when working with sepia, the ink from the cuttlefish. He made a potency of the ink and cured the artist of his complaints. The pure pigment is triturated to make the homoeopathic remedy.

Causation: Overlifting.

Worse: Cold air. Getting wet. Sitting, standing, kneeling. Before thunderstorms.

Better: Hard pressure. Violent exercise. Heat and warmth. Dancing.

Complaints: Achilles tendinitis and peritendinitis. Back pain and prolapsed disc.

Lower limbs: Achilles tendon feels too short. Legs restless and twitching. Feet feel cold.

Back: The pain comes on suddenly, as if struck by a hammer or kicked.

Lumbar and sacral pain is burning, tearing and throbbing. Spine rigid and very stiff. Dull ache in the lumbar spine, extending into the thighs. Sore to touch, but hard pressure relieves it. Stands with back pressed hard against something like a door jamb. Coughing hurts. Worse when sitting. Walking about eases the pain. History of back injury and weakness because everything affects the back. Bending forward is painful.

Mental/Emotional: Angry, sensitive, irritable, easily offended. Indifferent. Becomes offhand with close acquaintances. Strangely better from strenuous, even violent, exercise and dancing.

Silica

Silica is the most common mineral in the earth's crust. It comes in many forms and is found in most rocks. In the body it is a component of teeth, tendons, nails and hair. The remedy is made by trituration of crystals of silicon dioxide.

Causation: Injuries. Splinters.

Worse: Cold air, draught, damp, touch, pressure.

Better: Warm wrapping. Summer. Electrical treatments.

Complaints: Athlete's foot. Loss of confidence. Wounds. Scars. Bruised heel. Bruised toenail. Ankle sprains. Achilles tendon tears. Collateral ligament injuries. Prepatellar bursitis.

General Uses: Inflamed wounds, with splinters and material inside. Removes splinters and troublesome scars. To disperse scar tissue. and adhesions. Slow healing of cuts.

Lower limbs: Athlete's foot with cracks between the toes, slow inflammation, suppurative, itching and painful. Offensively smelly sweaty feet. Bruised, throbbing pain in heel which prevents walking, nails are rough, brittle, blue or black. Weak ankles and feet. Cramp in soles of feet. Bruised, throbbing pain in toe. Pain prevents walking.

Sticking pains and increased sensitivity to pain. Stiffness and pain from scarring to tissue. Chronically weak ankles and feet. Leg feels paralysed, cannot walk. Will remove scar tissue, and release adhesions. He may have rough, yellow, brittle nails.

Enlargement of the prepatellar bursa, and any inflammatory knee conditions. Paralysis of the legs when walking. Kneeling and pressure make it worse. Cramps in the calves in the evening after training.

Mental/Emotional: Loss of self-confidence in anticipation of an event. Afraid of failure and its consequences. Decides against performing, and nothing will shake that resolve. At other times is most cooperative and agreeable. Conflict between confidence and lack of it. After injury lacks determination and confidence to recover. Hides this feeling with obstinacy and a kind of determination.

Warning: The homoeopathic remedy is well known to cause the body to eject foreign objects, and should not be used when articles such as plates and screws have been used following injuries, or when the person has, for example, a pacemaker. A replacement hip or a polytetrafluoroethylene (PTFE) repair to a cruciate ligament may be rejected following Silica in higher potencies than the 6c.

Spongia Tosta

Powdered burned sea sponge was used in the Middles Ages for many complaints. The homoeopathic remedy is made from roasted sponge.

Worse: After sleep. Cold wind. Exertion. Tobacco. Excitement.

Better: Eating or drinking warm things.

Complaints: Cough.

General Uses: Very distinctive cough. Like sawing thin board. Rough, hollow and barking. Sensation of sponge, leaves or tissue in the larynx, and has to breathe through it. Voice is hoarse and the larynx painful dry and constricted. Breathing is deep, and loud between bouts of coughing. Fears asthma or some other serious illness.

Staphysagria

Delphinium staphysagria is a plant native to southern Europe. It was used externally for warts, lice and itching. It is said that the homoeopathic remedy, taken orally, discourages biting insects. The remedy is made from triturating the seeds.

Causation: Injury. Falls.

Worse: Stretching. Night.

Better: After breakfast.

Complaints: Cuts and lacerations. After surgery.

General Uses: This remedy has the reputation of healing cuts from sharp instruments, and has been prescribed for post operative care for many years. It also has a reputation for healing lacerated fibrous tissue.

Lower limbs: Knee feels beaten and painful after operation.

Sticta Pulmonaria

The English name for this plant is Lungwort, because the leaves have the appearance of lung tissue. Under the ancient 'Doctrine of Signatures' it was believed that the plant had the ability to cure inflammation of the respiratory tract. The whole plant is used to make the homoeopathic remedy.

Worse: Night. Breathing (cough). Lying.

Better: Sitting quietly.

Complaints: Bursitis. Injuries to bursae. Cough.

General Uses: Incessant, very dry, hacking cough that prevents sleep. Worse from lying in bed. Better for sitting quietly. Tickling high in the larynx. After colds, flu and long-term strenuous exertion.

Lower limbs: Bursitis in the knee. Swollen, stiff and painful with lancinating, rheumatic pain. Red, hot spots of inflammation in affected joints. Feet cold and damp. Injured and swollen bursae feel spongy and hot.

Mental/Emotional: Restlessness. Talks much, and does not care whether anyone listens. Floating feeling.

Strontium Carbonicum

Strontium carbonate. The remedy is made by trituration.

Worse: Cold. Walking. Sprains.

Better: Heat. Hot bathing.

Complaints: Ankles sprained and very puffy. Continued oedema long after injury in ankles and knees.

Lower limbs: Gnawing pain into the bones of the ankle and knee. Sprained and puffy ankles. Continued swelling long after injury with burning, gnawing pains. One limb feels immobile and weak.
Mental: Irritability, with sudden anger.

Sulphur

Sulphur is one of the substances ejected by volcanic eruption, and is otherwise known as brimstone. It occurs naturally and is an essential constituent of all living tissue. The homoeopathic remedy is one of the deepest acting and most commonly prescribed in the materia medica, with a wide range of actions.

In sports medicine, however, there are few specific applications for Sulphur. Many of your patients may nonetheless need it as a constitutional remedy. If you suspect this, please refer them to a qualified homoeopath.

The remedy is made from triturated pure sulphur or as a tincture by solution.

Causation: Sprains. Overexertion.

Worse: Warm bathing and applications. Being warm in bed. Exertion.

Better: Open air. Motion.

Complaints: Athlete's foot. Acute ankle sprain. Headache. Skin problems.

General Uses: Headache with nausea, comes on regularly every seven days, worse from standing and bathing. Hot and sweaty. Unwashed, untidy, unconcerned about his body odour which is there despite bathing. Spotty adolescent boys typify the kind of person needing Sulphur for their skin eruptions and general condition.

Lower limbs: Itching at night in bed. The feet are burning hot and must be put out of bed. Skin burns when scratched. Excoriation between the toes. Dirty feet. Skin around and between the toes is dry, rough and scaly. Violent and voluptuous itching. He cannot resist scratching and picking at his feet. Ankle swollen, stiff and feels heavy. Burning and stitching pains. Walks unsteadily. Dislikes standing.

Mental/Emotional: Untidy, talks about his theories, which may be outrageous and far-fetched. Lazy, hungry and always tired. Hopeful dreamer who loves to expound his theories and philosophy. Thinks mundane things are very beautiful. Talks late into the night.

Symphytum

This remedy is derived from the common plant known as comfrey, knitbone, knitback, bruisewort, boneset, healing plant and consolida. The name 'comfrey' comes from the Latin *con firma,* to form or unite. You may guess from these names that it has been used for a very long time in country and herbal medicine to cure broken bones and damaged tissue. The famous medieval herbalist, Culpeper, claims that if the leaves are boiled with separated pieces of meat in a pot, it will join them together again. The homoeopathic remedy is made from the chopped and pounded root whose juice is extracted after standing in alcohol.

Causation: Fractures, falls, blows, injuries.

Worse: Injuries. Blows from blunt instruments. Touch.

Complaints: Fractures and tears of all types, and from any cause. Injuries to eye and face.

General Uses: The remedy has uses in fractures, especially those that are slow and difficult to heal, and torn muscles, tendons and ligaments – it simply promotes fusion. Sore, bruised pain in eyeball after a blow.

Upper limbs: Following fractures and tears. Especially if they are slow to unite.

Lower limbs: Following fractures. Torn Achilles tendon. Meniscus and collateral ligament tears. Especially if they are slow to unite.

Back: Degeneration of the vertebrae.

Tellurium

Tellurium is an element found in combination with such metals as gold, silver and lead. The homoeopathic remedy is made by trituration.

Causation: Falls and injuries to the spine.

Worse: Touch, cold, lying on affected part.

Complaints: Injuries and blows to the sacrum.

Back: Blows, falls and injuries that affect the sacrum. The right side of the sacroiliac symphysis is affected, and pains extend down the right thigh. Soreness is the main complaint. Touch hurts so much that he fears it, and avoids it. Longstanding muscle spasm in the lumbosacral region. The back pain is worse on coughing or laughing.

Mental/Emotional: Fears being touched in sensitive places. Mentally excitable and touchy. Flies off the handle.

Thuja

The *Thuja occidentalis* tree is known as the white cedar, and grows in Mediterranean countries and North America. In ancient times the wood was burnt at sacrifices. The homoeopathic remedy is made from the leaves and twigs, gathered when the tree is flowering. They are pulped and allowed to stand in alcohol before the liquor is extracted and succussed.

This remedy is readily available in most health food stores and pharmacies, mainly because it is recommended for treating warts and verrucas. It is a deep-acting remedy, however, and ideally should be prescribed by a qualified homoeopath. Use it carefully for warts, and restrict it to one or two doses.

General Uses: Verrucas and warts. Cauliflower-shaped, especially when they are large, stinging and bleeding.

Urtica Urens

The common stinging nettle *Urtica dioica* has been used medicinally since ancient times. *Urtica urens* is its small brother. The homoeopathic remedy is made from the juice of the fresh plant picked in flower.

Causation: Burns. Stings. Blows.

Worse: Cool moist air, touch.

Complaints: Blisters. Grass burns. Burns. Sore lips.

General Uses: Stinging, burning blisters, worse from cold bathing and touch. This ointment is an excellent remedy for minor burns. Intense burning pain. Prevents blistering. Burned, sore, smarting lips from exposure to the sun.

Upper limbs: Continuous pain in the right deltoid, worse rotating the arm inwards.

Lower limbs: Acute gout with burning pain.

Variolinum

This remedy is prepared from lymph extracted from a smallpox pustule, triturated and potentised.

Causation: Blows and falls on the back.

Worse: Motion.

Complaints: Backache. Lumbar pain.

General Uses: Effects of falls and injuries to the lumbar spine and sacrum. Intolerable and excruciating pain extends down the legs, and into the abdomen. As if the back would break. Rising from a seat difficult and painful. Rheumatic pain in the muscles of the back. Any movement is painful. Very restless. Tosses and turns at night in bed. Looks tired and complains of lack of sleep.

ADVANCED USES OF HOMOEOPATHY
Chapter 11

Susceptibility to Injury

In this chapter I discuss the use of several very high potency remedies (1M and 10M) in circumstances affecting the mental and emotional condition of sports and dance performers. Although these potencies are safe, care must be taken when considering repeated doses. In my experience, a person who needs a remedy in high potency to counteract a negative 'mindset' will find that one or two doses will suffice to develop a more positive and confident attitude. If they do not, it is most likely that the remedy chosen was not the correct one. It is advisable, in all circumstances involving the possible use of high potencies, that the prior advice of a qualified homoeopath should be sought.

PREDISPOSITION TO INJURY

Why are some athletes or dancers more prone to injury than others? While it is possible to predict that more soccer players will suffer ankle and knee injuries than swimmers, and basketball players and cricketers will suffer more finger injuries than track and field athletes, we should also consider the whole question of predisposition to injury. We should ask ourselves whether certain types of persons may be predisposed towards certain injuries.

Many variables predispose an athlete to injury. Anatomical and biomechanical make-up, as well as a history of previous injury, age and sex, may all predispose an athlete or dancer to further injury. Objective tests have been used to study the phenomena of self-esteem, general personality, trait anxiety and locus of control. Relationships have been found between apprehension and injury. Being overprotective, easily distracted and attention-seeking may also predispose to injury. There may also be some connection between predisposition to injury and major life events such as bereavement, divorce, transfers and leaving home.

Homoeopathy is a very subjective system of medicine. At some levels of homoeopathic philosophy we believe that a person's worst fears and nightmares may be part of their dysfunctional vital force. It may be that the most severely disturbed vital force has the capability to lead the athlete or dancer towards fulfilling these. Injury disturbs the vital force and the whole person as soon as it happens. Perhaps this is why so many dancers and sports persons fear injury so deeply and also why they are susceptible to injury.

Anxiety

Anxiety plays an important part in predisposition to injury. It can cause abnormal behaviour in otherwise familiar, well-trained situations – risk-taking, overprotection and tension. A performer who is over-tense yet denies anxiety may be emotionally vulnerable and subject to loss of composure. The performance loses its intuitive quality, becomes awkward and results in injury. We have discussed performance stress in Chapter 7, and suggested remedies for anxiety and nerves in Chapter 9.

Guilt

Guilt is a familiar manifestation of anxiety that leads to self-punishment and confirmation of failure. A performer can feel guilty because he or she has not trained enough, because he has not achieved the goals set by himself, his parents, coach, manager, director or supporters. He may feel guilty because he has neglected his family to play this game, or thinks she is letting the company down, or indeed for very many different reasons. Guilt is a commonplace indulgence and a convenient excuse for poor performance.

Several homoeopathic remedies that have 'anxiety of conscience' or guilt as part of their symptom pictures. The best known of these is Aurum Metallicum, which is a very effective remedy when the person becomes depressed as a result of intense feelings of guilt.

Remedy Patterns

We have discussed in early chapters the patterns that homoeopaths recognise as being part of the picture we build up of our remedies. We believe it is no accident that the Calcarea Carbonica type of person suffers from repeated ankle injuries. Our materia medica describes the type and tells us that they have weak ankles. Nor is it any accident that the dancer who is anxious, dissatisfied and depressed with her performance regularly suffers tendon or ligament injuries, for this is the mental picture of Ruta. An astute and experienced homoeopath could probably forecast what injuries athlete or dancers will encounter simply from recognising the remedy patterns.

But it may be that the injury produces the pattern! There is an element of the 'chicken and egg' problem here. We recognise that susceptibility has a large part to play in injury, and it pays to note the mental patterns that exist.

A homoeopath is trained to regard psychological factors as indicators of a remedy. Depression, insecurity, indecision, jealousy, competitiveness, fulfilment and a desire to please are all commonly expressed in the confidential atmosphere of the homoeopathic consulting room, and can lead to a choice of remedy that has the power to turn such negative connotations into positive energy. The homoeopathic consultation should be without prejudice, based on observation, and with understanding of the pressures of the professional athlete or dancer.

LESSONS FROM THE WORLD OF DANCE

'Dancers are artists who are athletes, and athletes who are artists.'
(Fit to Dance)

There can be no question that professional dancers rank among the fittest and most dedicated of physical performers. It is among the most demanding forms of human movement and, as such, increases our knowledge of what the human body can achieve under stress. Although most dancers are injured as the result of fatigue and overwork, other psychological factors are perceived as playing a significant part in injury. Dancers suggest that depression, anxiety about performance and career and low self-esteem all precipitate injuries.

OTHER PSYCHOLOGICAL FACTORS

One of the more important studies of predisposition to injury was conducted by F. H. Sanderson. He suggests that the six main psychological factors are as follows:

Counterphobia
The athlete counters anxiety by being overaggressive and fearless, repeatedly testing his courage and indestructibility.

For example, a player may be so anxious that he loses control and behaves crazily. He is so disappointed at an important defeat that he cries openly. He laughs foolishly, sings, babbles and frequently gets into quarrels. He may strike, spit at or even kick another player in his excitement. He can be jealous and suspicious. A very sociable person, he dislikes being alone, likes to drink beer, but is often badly affected by drinking, and this leads him into trouble and to lose control. His injuries will come on suddenly, perhaps as the result of a sudden violent and thoughtless action. The pain will be sore and tearing.

I believe that giving the above player Hyoscyamus in a high potency, say 1M, for two days would reduce his chance of losing control and with it his susceptibility to injury.

Other people demonstrate counterphobia in other ways. If we can recognise the pattern and give them the appropriate remedy, their performances could be improved and the risk of injury reduced.

Masochism

This athlete or dancer has extremely high ambitions and works hard to achieve them. He has been determined to succeed from a very young age, trains hard, plays hard and thinks of little else. His parents are also ambitious and very supportive. He can be depressed, almost for no reason, but especially if he loses a match. He may enjoy music, walking and moonlight. He is motivated by guilt that he will not fulfil his own and his parents' ambition, and regards injury as a form of punishment. His knees are often painful and injured. The pains are deep in the bones and difficult to relieve.

Two or three doses of Aurum Metallicum in a high potency could relieve the need for masochism and guilt, strengthen the knees, relieve the bone pains, and could also make him feel less depressed and guilty.

Injury as a Weapon

To punish parents with high expectations, club, manager, coach or supporters.

A good example of this type is the athlete who is normally reserved and detached, seems insensitive to the feelings of others and may be perceived as arrogant. He takes offence easily and does not forget old hurts. He may seem resentful. He avoids consolation and sympathy. He is very careful about his possessions and worries in case they may be stolen. Because he does not forget grudges, but cannot overtly punish people like his parents or manager for them, the punishment is turned inwards in the form of injuries. These affect mainly the legs, knees and ankles. He may be very prone to hamstring injuries.

Give him three doses of one Natrum Muriaticum in high potency, 10M, over three days to reduce the susceptibility to injury.

Avoidance of Competition

The training-room athlete who cannot face the failure implied in competition, and who uses injury to opt out.

Duality

This person is full of conflict and seems to be two people, and cannot decide which one to be. One of them trains hard and seems to be determined to succeed at his chosen activity, with a fixed idea of where he is going. The other seems to lack the confidence to achieve his aims and predicts difficulties for himself. Although he loves training and works hard at it, he becomes exhausted and almost paralysed with tiredness. It is as if he lacks the power to perform. He suffers from muscle pains, tears, cramps, trembling, almost paralysis. His muscles tear easily, but what he suspects is a hamstring tear, for example, usually turns out to be a cramp.

Two or three single doses of Anacardium 10M spread over three days will help him to overcome his indecision.

Conflict

Another type is the person who is yielding and acquiescent at times, and at other times surprisingly obstinate and stubborn. He has fixed ideas about little things, and worries about them. He has an unfounded but real dread of failure. He loses his usual self-confidence. Everything becomes worse as he develops nervous excitement about a performance or match, and his loss of confidence develops into an injury. He has weak arms and shoulder, and injury may focus in his ankles and knees.

I would expect one dose of Silica 10M every day for three days to give this athlete or dancer more confidence. But, as ever, first note the warning about Silica on page 264.

Demonstration of Courage

The athlete who derives admiration or sympathy from bearing an obvious injury or scar. Two remedy types seem to fit this category.

The first enjoys stimulation and competition, is very energetic, and responds to any challenge. He can be angry, impatient, and irritable. He enjoys working at anything, and is worst when prevented from doing so. Bearing the scars of injury fulfils two purposes. Firstly, it justifies his lowered efficiency at work or training, and secondly it produces sympathy, which he relishes. Best of all it attracts attention to him, which he thoroughly enjoys. This is the ultimate 'no pain, no gain' athlete.

This person could benefit from one tablet daily for two days of Nux Vomica 10M.

The second type is mild and a little timid, craves sympathy, and feels much better when he has plenty of it. At other times she may be quite easily discouraged and can be tearful, crying easily for little reason. She loves being with people, and needs them for encouragement. Injury produces the sympathy she loves. She may cry a little when telling you about it.

Pulsatilla, one tablet of 1M for three days will probably benefit this person.

Psychosomatic Injury

For emotional or mental reasons the athlete makes more of his injury than is justified by its severity.

Homoeopaths do not differentiate between psychosomatic and other injuries when they consider the effects of injuries on people. We believe that any injury affects the whole person immediately it happens. Some people will be more sensitive to the mental and emotional effects than others. A remedy chosen according to the total symptom picture may help to reduce the effect of the physical injury.

Homoeopathic Equivalents

Homoeopathy was developed before the objectivity and language of modern psychology became familiar. Its terminology is subjective. As we treat every person as a unique individual we tend not to categorise them. Broadly objective terms such as masochism need to be translated into everyday language to be used to choose homoeopathic remedies.

Let us take the performer who denies anxiety, as an example. This person is fundamentally apprehensive, anxious and afraid of injury. He may weep, avoids sympathy and caring. He becomes angry and seems depressed and overexcited, but denies the tension and anxiety and says that there is nothing wrong. He forgets instructions and parts of his routine. Typically he will have to rush to the lavatory.

In Sanderson's terms this performer could be termed 'counter-phobic' or suffering from 'state anxiety'. In homoeopathic terms I would say he needs Arnica, and would give him one dose of the 1M potency before any competition or performance.

My reasons for this would be because the anxiety, fear of injury, resistance to sympathy and all those other denial symptoms are typical of Arnica, and the 1M potency tends to work on the psychological level more effectively than the lower potencies.

TREATING THE POTENTIAL FOR INJURY

Can we predict who is most likely to be injured and what the injury will be?

If you refer to Chapter 10, the materia medica for the homoeopathic remedies, you will see that each one contains a section on mental and emotional symptoms, and another on general symptoms. So far in this book we have used these as an aid to differentiate between the remedies recommended for physical injuries.

Every injury, however minor, has a wider effect on the organism than the tissue changes in the injured part. The sufferer is changed after injury. At the least, the effect is to make the person more careful of similar circumstances in future, to change his life in an empirical way. Every injury produces changes on mental, emotional and physical levels that must be taken into account when choosing the remedy. To ignore these other changes is to risk delaying recovery and to increase the susceptibility to injury in the future.

In other words, we have to consider the totality of the person's symptoms for even minor injuries. I would like to think that a homoeo-pathic remedy chosen according to a person's mental and physical symptoms would have the effect of helping that person to avoid injury. It would be interesting to explore this hypothesis as a research project.

TREATING THE WHOLE PERSON

If homoeopathic medicine is truly for the whole person, then a remedy prescribed for a physical injury will also cure the mental symptoms that accompany the physical injury. Thus, if we give someone Arnica for his bruising after a trauma, it should also make him less fearful of further injury and more accepting of treatment. One of the effects of giving Ruta to someone with a tendon injury should be to relieve his discontent and depression, and make him more positive towards recovery.

We can use the mental and general symptoms to forecast what to expect in the way of physical injuries and susceptibility. It may be possible to forecast how an athlete, dancer or performer will respond to injury, and choose remedies to anticipate that response. It should also be possible to reduce or remove the player or dancer's susceptibilities to injury completely and permanently. The correct constitutional remedy should do this.

This system involves knowing the athlete or dancer and the remedies, and being able to recognise that persons's constitutional remedy.

The remedy pictures in Chapter 10 and other literature may lead you to experiment with homoeopathy in this way. Although homoeopathic remedies have no side effects, they can be powerful medicines, and you should seek prior advice from a professional qualified homoeopath if you are in any doubt.

RESULTS OF INJURY

The mental and emotional responses of an athlete to injury are similar to most traumatic life incidents, and to the response when a person receives bad news. This may be similar to a grief response, with denial, anger and depression.

First there is denial, 'I'm OK. I'm fine. There's nothing wrong with me.' This is typically what the athlete first says. We have already met this often in this book when discussing Arnica. Serious injury can lead to post-traumatic shock. At this stage the athlete is unaware of severe pain or disability and the psychological effect is small.

Secondly, the initial denial response quickly turns to anger and dissatisfaction, and the athlete may express this against himself or others. Sometimes the anger turns against those closest to him. Then, as the athlete realises the seriousness of the injury and its likely effects, he becomes depressed. Perhaps he despairs of recovery.

Later, the psychological effects of serious injury can be considerable, and may lead the athlete to refuse treatment. Typically the responses are:

- Believing treatment and rehabilitation to be ineffective.
- Questioning the wisdom of the therapist because he thinks he is giving him the wrong treatment.
- Seeking other advice, perhaps visiting three or four other therapists.
- Believing the therapist is not interested in him and his injury.
- Failure to take responsibility for recovery and developing apathy towards rehabilitation.

Factors such as the history of previous injury and recovery, support systems, personality and the seriousness of the injury all influence the coping mechanism. Frequent injuries may lead the athlete or dancer to become frustrated and bitter.

These negative responses can be serious drawbacks to recovery, and any medication that can help avoid them would be useful. Several of the most frequently recommended homoeopathic remedies have strong indications for the psychological responses described above.

HOMOEOPATHIC REMEDIES FOR REACTION TO INJURY

The following descriptions are of some of the more common remedy patterns I have observed in active people. Further study of the remedy patterns, together with the injuries they are most susceptible to, could – perhaps – help you to take preventive action by giving them the remedy before they are injured. You should assess them according to the observed totality of symptoms of the athlete. If his pattern fits that of the remedy it will help his total recovery and prevent further injury. If you are uncertain about which remedy to choose, seek the advice of a qualified homoeopath.

Anacardium
The person typically exaggerates the seriousness of the injury and its effects. This becomes part of the inner conflict between determination to succeed and reach objectives and insecurity and a lack of confidence that makes difficulties and obstacles to success. There is a sense of duality about the person. At one time pleasantly absent-minded, under-confident and seeking reassurance; at another time impatient, angry and aggressively bad-tempered with a tendency to curse and swear. This

athlete or dancer will be susceptible to muscle cramps and tears, and may report a simple muscle spasm as a tear.

Dosage: One Anacardium 200c tablet will help to restore confidence and eliminate the tendency to exaggerate injury.

Arnica

This remedy is very strongly indicated when there is denial of injury and an insistence that he is well. This is followed by anger. He is very agitated, irritable and quarrelsome. His anger can turn to rage. He may shout and swear, and cry with frustration. He will be remorseful following an outburst of temper. He really fears being approached by others because they may touch him and cause further injury. He tends to be frightened and apprehensive and despairs of ever being able to play again. He may then become depressed and absent-minded, and finds concentration difficult. This is accompanied by so much anxiety about his recovery that you may think him hypochondriacal. After a head injury he may be apathetic and indifferent to external stimuli. Loss of memory after head injury may be marked.

Dosage: Arnica should be taken in the 30c, 200c or 1M potency for three or four doses following any traumatic serious injury.

Arsenicum Album

You may become conscious of the person who needs Arsenicum Album because he is so demanding, fastidious, fault-finding and oversensitive. Like Arnica, this person says that he is well when he is not, but not so markedly as in Arnica. He is much more angry about his injury, and may be violent. Then he becomes hopeless about recovery, depressed and irritable, and seeks other treatment and advice. He will consult many doctors and therapists. This is usually to confirm his own, very fixed ideas about his treatment. He is punctilious about being on time for appointments. His depression can lead to suicidal thoughts and thoughts of death. This can be a seriously depressed patient who should be referred to his GP or a qualified homoeopath. His injuries are frequent, and almost always produce burning pain for which he demands heat treatment.

Dosage: Arsenicum Album 1M, one tablet.

Bryonia

The person who needs Bryonia does not deny that he is injured, but is angry, morose and irritable about it. He is anxious about the future, despairs of being better, wants to be left alone to get on with being ill, and talks about poverty. He may be suspicious that he is not receiving the best treatment, and complains to the therapist over his treatment and time away from activity. Conversely he may become timid and very acquiescent as long as it means he will be left alone. You may observe a capricious approach to rehabilitation and recovery. Injury makes him reluctant to move.

Dosage: One Bryonia 1M tablet each day for three days.

Calcarea Carbonica

Think of this person as being flabby and disinclined to work towards rehabilitation on his own initiative. He nonetheless reads up about the medical details of his injury and condition. Of all your patients he despairs the most of getting better, and is the most reluctant to exercise. He does not want to be seen as injured or different. He may be abrupt in his attitude to others, and seem rough and ill-mannered, but this is merely a strategy to hide his embarrassment. He becomes very depressed during injury, forgets to attend your clinic and is irritable and suspicious. His weakness is focused in his ankles, wrists, and knees. Frequent sprains are inevitable. Most injuries will give rise to swelling.

Dosage: One Calc. Carb. 1M, three times on one day only.

Hypericum

Because Hypericum is more likely to be needed after an injury to nerve-rich regions, such as the base of the spine or following head injuries, there is likely to be less denial of injury and fear of being touched or approached. There may, however, be some euphoria and light-headedness – a feeling of floating. Injury follows an exceptionally successful performance, and you have a feeling that he reaches heights only to be brought down. He may seem excited and wants to be active even if his injury obviously prevents it. The pain soon becomes intolerable, and this brings anxiety, fright, anger, rage, fury and then despair. He is very sensitive to further pain. The pains make him depressed.

Dosage: One Hypericum tablet in the 200c potency.

Rhus Toxicodendron

This remedy is more likely to be needed from a day or two after injury to well into the rehabilitation period. Because the physical symptoms are better when the person is active and mobile we can expect the psychological symptoms to be aggravated when the person is inactive. All the mental symptoms are worse at night. He is morose, depressed and gloomy, restless, frustrated and sad, and all is worse after midnight when he is in bed. He may be irritable, yet strangely mild-mannered. Anxiety about his recovery is marked when he is at home in bed, and better when he is walking in the open air. He will be discouraged, and suspicious that he is not receiving the correct treatment or rehabilitation. Restlessness is very marked in this person. It is worst at night and disturbs his sleep. This restlessness is most evident in young people.

Dosage: One Rhus Tox. 1M tablet before bed for restlessness at night. It may be repeated as the symptoms demand, but the remedy must not be taken merely as a preventative.

Ruta Graveolens

Although this remedy is better known for its relationship to tendons and ligaments, I have known it work well on patients' depression following injury. It has seemed to encourage them to overcome their problems and to develop a more positive approach to their recovery. The person can be depressed and sad following injury, but the main component is his discontent and dissatisfaction with his injury and possibly his treatment. When not injured he can be dissatisfied with himself, irritable, morose and quarrelsome, and may be quite restless. Note that the symptoms of Ruta are not aggravated at night like those of Rhus Tox., and he is not as restless. One strange general symptom of this remedy is that he wakes from sleep with a start. Expect strained and injured tendons.

Dosage: One dose of Ruta 200c.

REFERRAL

There are many more homoeopathic remedies which can help the athlete or dancer to become less susceptible to injury, overcome the psychological effects of injury, and develop a positive attitude to rehabilitation. A qualified homoeopath will be able to discuss potential remedies with you, and to see patients who you consider may be helped by a deeper case analysis. See Appendix I for details of the registers of medical homoeopaths and professional homoeopaths.

Chapter 12

Enhanced Performance

'Scientists at Birmingham have begun a £95,000 investigation on the effects of intensive exercise and the possible damage to athletes' immunity to infection.' (*The Times*, 15 April 1996)

Although there is evidence that moderate physical activity enhances immune function, modern epidemiological data support the view that demanding, exhausting exercise increases the susceptibility to viral infection. Professional athletes in the weeks leading up to final competition, international cricketers, footballers and rugby players undertaking tours in the closed season approach levels of overtraining that may suppress the immune function. Dancers in demanding roles, underfunded productions and protracted tours face the same dangers.

When training is pushed to the limit, subclinical injuries in the working muscles become frequent and could increase the vulnerability to infection at other sites in the organism. Inhalation of polluted air can induce a similar response in the lungs. In some cases – dancers and gymnasts for example – the diet may fail to meet the demands of the exercise, and there is some speculation that this too reduces the immune response. The competitive professional athlete and performing dancer are exposed to high levels of psychosocial stress. Such stresses are likely to increase the vulnerability to viral infection.

I have no doubt that giving an athlete or dancer their constitutional remedy, just one dose at the start of a training or competition programme, will help increase their resistance to infections. It could promote a level of health that would enable them to undertake more strenuous and demanding training programmes than before, and to reach a higher standard of performance.

Recovery from hard, strenuous training schedules, intensive, prolonged and demanding performance, and long playing seasons can all be improved.

Apart from the physical effects of taking the constitutional remedy, the person's mental approach to training, competition, concentration and skills development can improve. Almost every case quoted in this book includes mental and emotional symptoms that contribute strongly to the choice of remedy.

Emotional preparation will be improved, as will the ability to cope with anxiety, nerves and anticipation during performance. Problems with irritability, sleeplessness, depression or indeed any emotional responses that interfere with performance can be overcome with the constitutional remedy.

The higher standards of mental, emotional and physical health can only contribute to better performance and more effective recovery.

MINIMISING THE RISK OF INFECTION

The sports physician or practitioner can recommend measures to reduce the likelihood of infection, such as minimising the exposure to pathogens, minimising psychological stress and taking care with the details of training and diet. At best these precautions can be 'hit or miss'.

While orthodox research spends time and money determining the causes of disease before a cure can be suggested, homoeopathic medicine simply takes the patient's symptoms and finds a remedy which fits as many of them as possible. Because it is an empirical and vitalistic medicine, the homoeopath does not have to rely on an orthodox diagnosis before prescribing. He can prescribe for the person as he is at the moment, and according to his previous symptom history. By taking an athlete's or dancer's case history and focusing especially on his mental, emotional, physical and general symptoms, the homoeopath can prescribe a constitutional remedy which, by improving the general level of health, will protect the person against the after-effects of a gruelling training and competition programme.

CASE 32

An international kayak competitor and team captain whose full-time job is in sports and recreation management suffered from vomiting and diarrhoea for some days after his return from major international championships at the culmination of his competition season. He could not drink even water or milk without vomiting. His abdomen felt distended, he had a lot of wind and noisy offensive flatus, a twisted pain in his abdomen and occasional diarrhoea which relieved the pain and nausea.

He felt as if his body had slowed down and that he could not get it going again. He felt extremely tired and as if any exercise would make him worse. He had stopped training and taking any exercise at all. Even daily chores had become too much for him. Bright sun made him feel sleepy. Almost everything made him tired and want to sleep. He had been invited to another competition, but turned it down because he felt so drained.

His work was not a problem because it helped him to forget his tiredness and nausea. Time passed too quickly; he wanted to be able to stand back and take stock of his life.

A new baby meant disturbed nights, which did not help the situation. He was a vegetarian because he had disliked meat since his teenage years.

He dreamed repeatedly of putting things in order to avoid upsetting people, and of stairs leading to darkness. He had started having nightmares of running about in a panic. He woke from them howling with fright.

He liked his daily life to be well ordered and to have things in their right place. He was always careful about security, and would double-check that everything was locked up before leaving home. He enjoyed organising training programmes, diet and schedules. At work he had two jobs and was also involved in coaching. He had a reputation for talking all the time, but his wife complained that when he got home he became uncommunicative and broody. He said that after training, competition or work he felt he needed time to unwind, and sat quietly to do this.

For this active, high-achieving international athlete his present state was a personal disaster, and he felt desperate.

Prescription

Two symptoms led me to a prescription. Both of them have the chosen remedy as the only one listed for that symptom, which is an almost certain sign of the correct remedy. They were both mental symptoms – He dreamed of running around in a panic and awoke howling with fright.

The only remedy for both these was Veratrum Album. I found that many more of his symptoms also fitted this remedy so I gave him Veratrum Album 30c once daily for two days. One week later he phoned to say he was feeling much better, the diarrhoea and vomiting had stopped almost immediately, and that his energy levels had increased. He had stopped working so hard, started exercising, and was looking forward to competing again.

IMPROVING PERFORMANCE WITH THE CONSTITUTIONAL REMEDY

I suggest in Chapter 11 that giving athletes the remedy which most nearly fits their mental and general pattern could prevent further injury or, indeed, prevent them being injured at all. Giving a person their constitutional remedy could also lead to improved performance.

My experience as a homoeopath and active sportsman has been that taking the constitutional remedy improves sustained tolerance to stress and improves affective regulation. These firstly enable the person to perform a chosen activity at a sustained high level, and, secondly, allow him to maintain a normal emotional balance while doing so. The advantage of these for any physical performer must be obvious.

Regardless of whether or not a person is manifesting acute disease, the constitutional remedy can ensure that the vital force keeps the organism in harmony, and will have positive effects on that person. It will enable him to undertake long-term and demanding performance without adverse effects. It will also prevent the deterioration of the immune system following such sustained activity.

A word of warning is appropriate. A person's vital force can also demand that the organism is rested, either physically or mentally. A deep-acting constitutional remedy will make the athlete more aware of his needs on all levels, and he may not be able to exercise demands on his body that will result in damage. In many ways this can be regarded as a sign of health.

A constitutional remedy should be taken under supervision and with care.

Responses to Stimuli

A person's constitutional remedy can change in response to stimuli. Trauma, vaccination, grief, loss and other influences can change the level at which an organism responds to the outside world and to imbalances from within. As these changes occur, so the vital force responds with different sets of symptoms, the totality of which can suggest a different constitutional remedy. This will be related to the originally perceived constitutional remedy. The skill of the homoeopathic practitioner lies in being able to recognise a person's constitutional remedy and the changes that occur to the organism in response to stress. From those changes he may decide to prescribe a new remedy or to change the potency of the current remedy.

PRACTICAL APPLICATIONS

Fatigue

Some remedies are well known for their effect of delaying the onset of fatigue and aiding recovery from exercise. Use them with care because it is possible that the vital force can respond by insisting that the organism rests immediately and for as long as it needs to recover. I have known someone given Arnica for his tiredness to fall asleep immediately. He woke one hour later, full of life and thoroughly recovered. The following remedies will help prevent fatigue:

Arnica

Every participant in long distance endurance events of any sort will benefit from taking one tablet of Arnica 30c before and after the event, and at any time that he feels exhaustion coming on during the event. It will delay the onset of fatigue and promote recovery. Typically the person who will respond best to Arnica is the one who denies he needs it and says he feels fine.

Dosage: One Arnica 30c before and after an event, and at any time it is needed.

Coca

This remedy is especially useful for exhaustion and fatigue generated by performing at altitude, but will also work at sea level. Mental and physical prostration from exertion. Exhaustion is mostly felt in the muscles. The mental prostration can alternate with a sense of exhilaration. There may be a loss of the sense of right and wrong. If an athlete who is given to silly and irrational lapses in behaviour at sea level intends competing above about 5,000 feet he should take Coca before doing so. It will prevent fatigue, and may help his control.

Dosage: One Coca 6c, followed by one Coca 30c when needed, and one Coca 200c at any time it is needed. This combination should not be repeated until some days have elapsed after the event and the athlete or dancer has rested and recovered.

At altitude give one Coca 30c before the first event, and repeated as necessary until the athlete feels fully acclimatised to altitude.

Piper Methysticum

One dose of this remedy has the ability to enable a person to exercise without fatigue. More than two doses will produce intense torpor and tiredness. It should only be used if the athlete or dancer is exhausted yet needs absolutely to continue. The person who will respond best to Piper Methysticum is someone who is highly strung and excitable, cheerful, enjoys dancing and entertainment, and eats hurriedly. Then suddenly he becomes bored, solitary, irritable, dull and sleepy, seemingly without cause. He has a headache, is restless, very sleepy during the day but sleepless at night, and very weak.

Dosage: One Piper Methysticum 6c when it is needed. Do not repeat!

Combination Remedy: Calcarea Phosphorica, Magnesia Phosphorica and Kali Phosphoricum

These three low potency remedies in combination have the reputation for increasing awareness, response to stimuli and endurance. The combination can be so powerful that it must be followed by another tissue salt, Natrum Phosphoricum, to enable the athlete to calm down and rest following the event.

Dosage: Calc. Phos., Magnesia Phos. and Kali Phos., all in the 6x potency: one of each before an event or performance. Follow this by Natrum Phos. 6x when the event is over.

Anxiety and Stress

A certain amount of anxiety before a performance is essential. The acceptable level of anxiety for each athlete or performer is a uniquely individual matter, but no-one performs well unless they are nervous. It is the high state of arousal generated by the big occasion that produces the great performance. When there is insufficient anxiety the performance may not reach the athlete's optimum level.

There is, however, a price to be paid for overarousal. Overanxiety depresses performance. When the anxiety becomes too much for the athlete, then there is a significant deterioration. Personal expectations and ambitions, and the expectations of family, coaches, sponsors and the public, the additional, stresses of long-term competition (for example a long cricket tour), minor injuries, the stress of high-level competition, jet lag and loss of sleep can all contribute to anxiety, reaching proportions which cause a drop-off in performance. Stage-fright before an important performance is often experienced by dancers.

Mental and Emotional Balance

The successful person functions in a balanced way which enables them to achieve a level of stress that stimulates better performance. This balance is the same as that achieved by a healthy vital force. The organism is capable of functioning at its highest potential on all levels without adverse effects to the organism. It is a sign of imbalance when the athlete or dancer succumbs to overanxiety or infection after a long and strenuous competition or training programme.

Assessing and prescribing the constitutional remedy will enable the vital force to maintain its balance under even the most strenuous circumstances. This will be the best remedy for overanxiety.

Artistic Performance

A dancer's performance is not only physical. It is essentially expressive, artistic, interpretative and controlled. Performance demands that the dancer prepares with relaxation, meditation and mental preparation for the predominantly artistic elements of the performance. Many dancers, however, report panic attacks on stage, blanking-out in performance, being unable to move or else a sensation as if wading through glue. A remedy that helps the dancer overcome the anxiety and nerves should help with the artistic element of performance.

Remedies for Anxiety

There are a few remedies that have the reputation for calming anxiety, especially in anticipation of an ordeal. Taken with care, they should improve performance by reducing tension and increasing the potential for relaxation.

Warning: Although they do not have side effects and cannot be detected by conventional drug tests, these powerful medicines can sometimes work too effectively and reduce anxiety to below optimum levels. Coaches and performers should work together to find exactly the right level of remedy and dosage for the best results. It is very difficult to 'self-prescribe' homoeopathic remedies successfully for essentially mental and emotional problems or symptoms such as anxiety. One has to be objective when choosing the remedy, and it would be advisable to consult a qualified homoeopath in these circumstances.

Argentum Nitricum

For the athlete or dancer who is nervous, impulsive, hurried and anxious. Dreads ordeals, and fears impending failure. Imagines minor illnesses. Imagines accidents and injuries vividly. Visualises them. Nervous headache. Anxiety affects the digestive system and performance. Diarrhoea before an event. It may be frequent, immediately after eating or drinking. Active thoughts prevent sleep. Sleep is very restless with horrid dreams. Craves sugar and sweets.

Dosage: One Argentum Nitricum 200c the night before, and one an hour before an event.

Arsenicum Album

Anxiety in response to expectations of others. Becomes breathless, weak and restless. Cannot live up to expectations, and becomes full of fear and nervousness as a result. This person is obsessive about routine and very superstitious about everything being exactly right. Has a reputation for fastidiousness, and may exasperate other people by demands that everything is exactly right. Very restless. Moves from place to place, chair to chair, or bed to bed. Sleep is disturbed and anxious. Gets up and moves around. Trembling in limbs with nervousness. Very thirsty for sips of cold drinks. May be sick with anxiety.

Dosage: One Arsenicum Album 200c the night before, and one an hour before an event.

Carcinosin

This remedy is almost a specific one for dancers. Anxiety increases with each event or performance, and experience does little to resolve it. The long-term buildup of excitement and anticipation results in a final attack of uncontrollable anxiety and nervousness, and a feeling of having lost control over the senses. Self-confidence disappears. Support and kind words worsen the state, and he avoids conversation. Fears failure, yet is convinced that he will fail, and suffers from inner conflict. A notoriously bad sleeper, not only before an event. More fastidious about details, cleanliness and punctuality (especially) than Arsenicum Album, but less concerned with routines. An athlete or dancer whose achievements are the culmination of long preparation by parents and coach since childhood. Conscious of the effort and cost of their training.

Dosage: One Carcinosin 200c a few days before an event.

Gelsemium

Overanxiety causes the muscles to become weak, tired, heavy and un-coordinated. The motor nerves are affected, causing loss of function and tension during normally relaxed and intuitive actions. The athlete or dancer may become totally relaxed to the level of prostration. Too anxious to perform at all. Urinates frequently and feels better. Really dreads the event. Wants to be left alone and quiet. Becomes solitary. Answers questions very slowly, as if in a daydream. Brooding and worried. Develops flu-like symptoms; cold, shivering, heavy-eyed, aching joints, in anticipation of event or performance.

Dosage: One Gelsemium 200c the night before, and one an hour before an event.

DEVELOPMENTAL REMEDIES

Very little research has been done into the effects of homoeopathic remedies specifically for improving athletic or other physical performance. The argument that a person's constitutional remedy will enable him to reach a higher level of fitness and health, and thus enable him to develop to his optimum level, is a valid one. But sometimes one needs more specific suggestions for improving performance. Any research into homoeopathic remedies for enhancing performance will inevitably result in anecdotal evidence, because remedies will only work when most of the individual's symptoms, physical, mental and emotional, most nearly match those of the remedy. This point is exemplified in the following case.

CASE 33

An 18-year-old rugby player came to me because of his ankle injury. He seemed to suffer frequent sprains. He looked big and strong, 6 ft tall and weighing 200 pounds. He worked hard at skills training and never missed a training session. His strength and power were much less than his build suggested, and his muscles were soft and lacking tone. It was as if his build belied his actual musculature. His playing performance was disappointing. He lacked stamina and never reached his promised potential. He seemed to suffer a drop-off in energy towards the end of matches. He told me he liked to eat eggs but was otherwise a vegetarian. His favourite food was sweets and puddings, but he disliked rice pudding because of the milk.

His coach described him as 'flabby'. He always trained below his capacity. He was fair-haired and fair-skinned. His handshake was surprisingly soft and flabby. He could be obstinate at times and take offence at slight remarks, and then would sit alone and sulk.

Comment

From his mental and general physical symptoms it was obvious to me that this player needed Calcarea Carbonica in a high potency. He was soft and flabby, fair, obstinate and easily offended, and liked eggs. He also had weak ankles that sprained easily.

His parents were both large, fair, slow-moving and had flabby hand-shakes. They were very supportive of their son's rugby ambitions.

I gave him Calc. Carb. 1M, two doses to be taken over twenty-four hours. His ankle recovered quickly and after two months the coach reported that his game had improved. He seemed stronger and fitter. The following season he was a changed player. His body shape had firmed up. He was certainly stronger and more able to use his strength. His speed around the field had improved, and he had lost his flabbiness. He went on to play at a good standard and realised his potential.

I am reluctant to claim that the homoeopathic remedy was entirely responsible for this player's changes. It probably had a part to play in it. The case demonstrates how the appropriate remedy can affect the person as a whole, and also have specific effects.

If a person generally fits the description of Calcarea Carbonica, with flabbiness, sweating, slowness and lack of physical and mental stamina, he will probably also fit some of the mental and emotional symptoms. Caucasians who fit this remedy will usually be fair-skinned and fair-haired. The remedy, if it is correct, will stimulate development on all levels and restore the balance of the individual's health.

A person does not need to be overtly ill for a remedy to work. I believe that the correct constitutional remedy can work positively to stimulate higher levels of health and physical and mental performance.

Here are some suggestions for remedies and other products that may be effective, as well as legal to use, to enhance performance and development of strength and power.

Arnica
Dosage: It is suggested by some homoeopaths that Arnica 6c taken regularly, about once a week for four weeks, will aid muscular development.

Calcarea Carbonica
Especially for fair, flabby persons with a slow metabolism who need to improve their strength, speed, power and endurance.
Dosage: One Calcarea Carbonica 30c weekly for two weeks.

Calcarea Phosphorica

This remedy, in the 6x potency, is said to improve the assimilation of proteins and promote the development of muscles, tendons and ligaments. It may be especially useful for athletes and dancers who have outgrown their strength and have undertaken training programmes that have been too strenuous or demanding. Young people who have grown to be tall, thin, scrawny and delicate as the result of overwork or overstudy. They may be peevish, restless and fretful, and want to travel.

Dosage: Take Calcarea Phosphorica 6x one tablet daily for two to three weeks.

Plumbum Metallicum

This remedy affects the muscles, enabling them to strengthen and develop. Better for hard massage and stretching. May be a quiet and remote person who is disinclined to talk much. Exertion and training make him weary.

Dosage: One Plumbum 30c daily for two weeks.

Sulphur

Homoeopathic Sulphur has the potential to increase the assimilation of nutrients in the body. It will counter weakness in individuals who tend to be untidy, always tired, and dreamers. Exertion tires them more than expected. Hot feet at night, which have to be pushed out of bed.

Dosage: One Sulphur 30c daily for two weeks.

If you intend trying any of the above over a period of more than two weeks, it is advisable that you should first consult a homoeopath for advice.

Chapter 13

Other Complementary Therapies and Techniques

The concept of whole health, as generated by holistic medicine, is a relatively recent idea in Western civilisation. You may have been persuaded by now that homoeopathy works with the whole person and that it is a holistic and vitalistic branch of medicine. There are also other complementary therapies which are applicable to specific injuries, as well as having the potential to improve general health and promote relaxation, relief of stress and performance. Sometimes the choice is bewildering for a sports person or dancer seeking to resolve an injury or its results.

I have compiled the following short list of those complementary therapies which, in addition to homoeopathy, I have seen to be effective, or which I have used in my own pursuit of fitness and health.

Warning: Elsewhere in this book I have warned about the dangers of self-diagnosis. It is essential to obtain an early medical diagnosis of any persistent condition. If a complementary therapy should then be preferred, it is no less important to choose a properly qualified practitioner of that therapy.

ACUPUNCTURE AND ACUPRESSURE

The principle of holistic medicine has provided the basis for Chinese medicine for many centuries. The Chinese recognise that mind and body are inseparable, both in sickness and health, and that all parts of an organism are connected and interdependent. Chinese medicine is wide-ranging, and acupuncture forms only one of its therapies.

Acupuncture is based on the belief that the body contains channels or 'meridians' through which the life force or 'Qi' (pronounced 'chi') flows and functions. Qi provides energy, control and balance for the organism and flows without interruption in the healthy body. If any part of the body is suffering from an injury or other disorder, the flow in the

293

relevant meridian will be diminished or interrupted. This disturbs the body's balance and causes illness, both in the injured organ and elsewhere.

There are surface points on the meridians, where, if needles are inserted, the nerves of the autonomic nervous system are stimulated. The impulse goes to the lower centres of the brain and then back again to the injured or diseased organ.

In terms of orthodox physiology this theory sounds almost as improbable as homoeopathy. It is possible, however, that the life force does operate through such channels. If the needles are inserted in the correct meridians they may stimulate the Qi. Countless thousands of cases prove the efficacy of acupuncture, and there are now many doctors using the techniques as part of their daily practice. Referral for acupuncture from a general practitioner has become commonplace.

Treatment

The acupuncturist's examination consists of detailed observation; looking, touching, smelling and asking. His main diagnostic tool is, however, his pulse-taking. This is an extremely complicated and fine skill that takes years to develop. There are twenty-eight basic types of pulse to feel and assess on the two wrists, and they give information that may be quite incomprehensible to westerners. The result is to trace the disharmony present in the patient.

Having diagnosed the complaint, the acupuncturist is faced with choosing from over one thousand points on fourteen meridians where he may place his needles. The practitioner's skill lies in selecting the points he knows will resolve this disharmony and stimulate the healing process.

Obviously, when preparing to stick needles into someone, the acupuncturist needs to be accurate and confident. Training, experience and qualifications lead him to know exactly where the insertion will be most effective. Various ways of stimulating these sites have been tried, and found to be more or less successful. Suction cups over sites, electric and sonic stimulation, heat and chemicals have all been used, with or without needles.

The actual experience of acupuncture is not as alarming as it sounds, providing that the therapist is properly trained and qualified. The needles are of the fineness of hair. On average only five to fifteen are inserted, and the patient reports no more than a faint pinprick on insertion.

Acupressure

One simple and effective method available to the lay person is acupressure, pressure being applied by the fingers on particular points to ease aches, pains, tension and fatigue. In this technique the pressure is applied over the appropriate acupuncture points – these can be located anywhere from a quarter of an inch to two inches below the surface, and require different pressure techniques. Fingers, thumbs or knuckles can be used. The points are up to a centimetre in diameter and are specific in area. As a general rule the specific acupressure point is more sensitive than the surrounding area, and if stimulation of a point becomes painful it should be discontinued. A sense of electrical stimulation following the course of a nerve radiating from a pressure point is, however, beneficial.

OSTEOPATHY

Osteopathy was developed in 1876 by an American physician, Dr Andrew Taylor Still, who began by studying the mechanical functioning of the body. He arrived at the belief that the structure of the body governs its function in all respects. Modern osteopaths have largely diverted from Still's belief that any disease can be cured by spinal manipulation, and concentrate more on the relief of back pain, joint and mechanical problems. It is a common experience that a patient who consults an osteopath for back pain will also experience relief of deeper conditions. I have also seen patients who have benefited generally from a combination of homoeopathy and osteopathy.

Osteopaths are skilled practitioners who deal with acute and chronic pain every day, treating over five million people a year in Britain. They are trained to recognise and treat many causes of pain, not only those originating in spinal lesions. The therapy is recognised by the British Medical Association as a discrete clinical discipline. Osteopathy has now become the first major complementary health care profession to be accorded statutory regulation in the UK. Many osteopaths work in conjunction with National Health Service general practices, and it is also possible for a doctor to refer a patient to an osteopath on the NHS.

Examination and Treatment

The osteopath will observe your overall posture and gait, looking for asymmetries or restrictions of mobility.

He or she will then take a detailed medical history before putting the patient through a thorough physical examination, during which any points of weakness, excessive strain or specific injury will be identified. A musculoskeletal assessment will be considered together with lifestyle factors and habitual physical tendencies.

The case-taking will often elucidate causes of misalignment, such as the runner who develops a pelvic tilt by always running the same way round a track, or regularly on a cambered road.

The osteopath will be able to use a number of methods to reduce inflammation, ranging from massage of soft tissue to manipulation and movement of joints. This helps to reduce muscle spasm and increase mobility, creating an environment which allows tissue to heal.

He will also be looking for areas of tension that can be eliminated by the gentle manipulation of joints, muscles and tendons to restore a full range of movement. Later, more vigorous manipulation may be employed. Some patients report that this vigorous manipulation produces a loudly audible sound, and may fear that they will be stretched and wrenched into painful positions. The 'sharp crack' that the patient may hear sounds much worse to him than it really is.

There may be some reactive discomfort after manipulation, and one may want to recommend a homoeopathic remedy to relieve it. I have often prescribed Hypericum 30c in a single dose in those circumstances. Your osteopath will also be able to recommend self-help methods of pain reduction to use at home.

CHIROPRACTIC

The founder of chiropractic, Daniel David Palmer, believed that the spine is of overriding importance in the health of the body. He discovered this system by curing the deafness of a patient with a sudden thrust to a misplaced vertebra. It is conceivable that misplaced vertebrae could press against nerves controlling almost every aspect of the body's function. Palmer founded a school of chiropractic in 1910, and developed a fresh approach to the art of spinal manipulation.

Chiropractors are fully trained to carry out spinal diagnosis and therapy at a sophisticated and refined level, and are becoming accepted by the orthodox medical profession as partners in the general health care system.

Despite this, and the benefits that thousands of patients derived from his care, Palmer was jailed for practising medicine in the United States without a licence, and thousands of prosecutions were instigated against chiropractors. Public outcry, however, succeeded in freeing these therapists, and by 1960 chiropractic was recognised as a *bona fide* therapy in most of the United States.

Sports injuries often create stresses on the spine which may cause misalignment, and overuse conditions can be generated by spinal misalignment. It is possibly more difficult to accept that almost all illness, including certain kinds of sports injuries, could result from spinal lesions or subluxations, and that by eliminating those lesions and subluxations the injury or illness may be cured.

Examination and Treatment

The chiropractor will make a detailed examination of the spine, feeling for any displacement. He will normally make any adjustments necessary immediately, often with dramatic results. Many chiropractors now use a diagnostic technique called 'applied kinesiology', which is a way of using systematic muscle techniques to assess physiological disturbances. Many also use X-rays for diagnosis.

The chiropractor will then usually apply a 'rapid, low impact, high velocity manual thrust' applied directly to a spinal lesion or fixation. This has the effect of releasing the joint and restoring it to its normal range of movement. Other techniques producing other different effects are also used, including deep massage, stretching and separating muscles to reduce, for example, muscle spasm.

Some patients report that this vigorous chiropractic manipulation produces a loud sound, and fear that they may be stretched and wrenched into painful positions. As in osteopathy, the 'sharp crack' sounds much worse to the patient than it really is.

Although many people regard as chiropractic as being a spinal therapy and seek their treatment mainly for the relief of lower back pain, my personal experience is that a chiropractor can relieve serious joint and other pain arising from injury, and thus promote effective recovery.

Principal Differences Between Osteopathy and Chiropractic

Osteopaths make more use of mobilising joints and use more soft tissue techniques than chiropractors. Traditionally the difference between these two manipulative techniques has been that osteopaths use greater leverage, whereas chiropractors use less leverage and more direct technique. An osteopath will often make contact some distance from the joint being manipulated; a chiropractor will use leverage directly over the vertebrae being adjusted.

HEALING

In Britain, healing has more practitioners and more patients than all other therapies combined. It is probably the most difficult of all the therapies to explain, yet it is the most readily accepted by orthodox medicine. Many GPs regularly refer patients to healers, usually at the patient's request. Many doctors also practise healing. Members of the National Federation of Spiritual Healers are permitted to work in hospitals. It may have some relevance in sports injuries, especially for recurring and chronic conditions.

Despite being almost inextricably linked with spiritualism or religious belief, many healers are reluctant to be known as 'faith' or 'spiritual' healers, and religious belief is not essential for patients to benefit. The healer often believes that his powers are derived from a superior being, and will only be able to work when those powers are 'available'.

The energy experienced by western healers may be similar to the 'Qi' experienced in Qi Gong, acupuncture and other Chinese health and healing systems. It is often reported as a feeling of intense heat generated by the healer's hands.

It is very likely that a healer could help promote the recovery of an injured athlete. It would probably depend on the attitude of the athlete, and his acceptance of the healer's craft.

QI GONG

Qi Gong, pronounced 'chi gong', is a Chinese healing and health-promoting art that dates back several thousand years. Archaeologists in China have discovered documented records of postural and breathing exercises that were practised to promote health. This system of training and exercise may be considered a sister to acupuncture, in that it uses the same energy meridians that maintain the function of the body. In the case of Qi Gong breathing techniques, postures and exercises are used to stimulate the Qi field in the body to enhance the quality of life and promote healing after injury.

One of the effects of traumatic injury is that the blood supply to the injured part is disrupted or interrupted. Many orthodox methods of treatment are designed to increase that blood supply.

One description of the Qi is that it is a stream of electrochemical energy that flows through the meridians to service the skin, muscles, ligaments, tendons, skeleton and organs. Where there is an abundance of qi there will also be an abundant blood supply.

The effects of Qi Gong therapy can be observed through the skin and eyes. The Chinese regard the former as an organ that demonstrates the health of the organism. A smooth healthy skin develops through increased lung capacity and breathing techniques, and strengthening of the 'Wei Qi', the external protective energy field. This is similar to the 'aura' that healers experience. The eyes become clearer and brighter.

When a joint is damaged, inflammation makes the skin appear red and feel hot. Later it may become pale, cold and discoloured from bruising. These two effects demonstrate the Chinese principle of yin and yang. These may be translated as yin being 'soft, cool, feminine' and yang being 'hard, hot, masculine'. Every movement, indeed everything living, is either yin or yang. Every injury and its effect is one or the other, or even both together.

The key features that make Qi Gong unique are the following:

- Postural corrections, biomechanical engineering.
- Enhanced breathing consciousness throughout the body.
- Application of 'yin' and 'yang' philosophy.
- Taoist principles of natural living.
- Repetition of treatment and exercise.

As it is the patient's own Qi that promotes the healing process – not that of the therapist – all the above principles must be adhered to and followed closely under the guidance of a skilled Qi Gong teacher.

When presented with an injury, the Qi Gong therapist will always check whether the patient has been diagnosed by a medically qualified practitioner, and that his Qi Gong treatment has that person's approval. A thorough examination follows, paying particular attention to joint function, skin condition, discoloration, swelling, heat, coolness and sensitivity. Massage and manipulation may follow, according to the yin or yang nature of the joint. The limb will be placed in the best position to open up Qi channels, and the patient advised on exercises.

A combination of rest and gentle movement would be prescribed to stimulate the Qi, especially in the injured limb, and keep the joint mobile. This will help reduce the time necessary for a return to normal function.

Qi Gong and Tai Chi exercises are excellent for maintaining joint mobility and warming up before dance, sports events or training – as well as for developing balance in all senses and for learning to 'centre' oneself. I can recommend them thoroughly from personal experience. Anyone wishing to maintain total body function, joint mobility, flexibility and good health would do well to seek out a Qi Gong and Tai Chi teacher.

REFLEXOLOGY

Reflexology is a method for activating the healing powers of the body by manipulating reflex areas in the feet. In the early years of the twentieth century Dr William Fitzgerald developed the zone theory of the body, arguing that parts of the body related to other parts. He demonstrated that by applying pressure to one area he could anaesthetise another. A physiotherapist, Eunice Ingham, concluded in the 1930s that since zones exist throughout the body, some areas may be more accessible and effective than others. She discovered that the feet were the most responsive for working all the zones, and then mapped the entire body onto the feet.

It was realised that alternating pressure on the various points had therapeutic effects far beyond the limited use to which zone therapy had previously been applied, and that it could effectively be used for the reduction of pain.

Energy Zones

As with acupuncture, acupressure, Qi Gong and Tai Chi, reflexology recognises the presence of the intangible life energy called Qi. Reflexologists specify that there are ten energy zones that run the length of the body from head to toe. All the organs and parts of the body lie along one or more of these zones or meridians.

Stimulating or 'working' any zone in the foot, by applying pressure with fingers or thumbs, affects the entire zone throughout the body. Working the kidney area on the foot will release energy through that entire meridian or zone and would, for example, revitalise and balance the function of the eyes – which lie in the same zone.

An important function of reflexology for sports persons and other performers is that its use can reduce stress and induce deep relaxation. Circulation proceeds smoothly, blood flow is improved, and oxygen reaches all the cells more efficiently. The nervous system calms down and functions more normally.

Technique

To begin to use reflexology it is necessary to study the art in depth. There are some techniques which may be useful to athletes and dancers to relax and stimulate parts of the body that are susceptible to injury and strain.

The most useful of these is 'thumb walking'. This is done with the outer edge of the thumb that touches a table when you lie your hand palm down on a table. The other four fingers grip the back of the foot and support the thumb. The thumb is bent at the first joint in contact with the sole of the foot, and takes a 'bite'. The release of the grip pushes the thumb forward in a small movement which 'walks' it up the foot. It is the bending movement that actually walks the thumb forward. The smaller the step the better.

Benefits

By making reflexology part of regular training, an athlete should improve strength and balance, suffer fewer injuries, and recover from those injuries he does receive. Seriously competitive athletes are not recommended to receive reflexology on the day of a competition, because the deep relaxation may reduce the tension level necessary for peak performance. A twenty-minute session will help athletes or dancers relax and recover after an event, and is useful in long and protracted competitions.

Reflexology is very useful for aching and injured muscles. The appropriate area of the foot should be stimulated by thumb walking after firstly relaxing and stimulating the whole foot. It can be used to relieve pain anywhere, and can stimulate the repair of broken bones and damaged ligaments.

Major injuries and chronic conditions can benefit from reflexology, but they require the skills and experience of a qualified practitioner.

ALEXANDER TECHNIQUE

Although the Alexander Technique is much more than simply a system for improving posture and breathing, its value in sports performance lies largely in just these aspects. It is a method of becoming more aware of one's body during everyday activities, and indeed all physical activities. More than this, it enables one to become more aware of the tensions that arise from mental postures such as anxiety, tension and stress.

An Alexander teacher will enable someone to release tensions that have gone unnoticed for months or years, and which may have become the triggers of aches and pains that accumulate with age. Although the main focus of the Alexander Technique is on the relief of back pain, adjusting the posture can relieve tension and pain, for example, in a shoulder suffering the long-term effects of a rotator cuff tear, or in a case of chronic ankle pain.

History

Frederick Matthias Alexander was born in Australia in 1869. He eventually became an actor who specialised in one-man recitations of Shakespeare. He was dismayed to find his career terminated by losing his voice, and made a study of his own postural stresses and tensions. He found that he tended to pull back his head, increasing the tension in his cervical area, depressing his larynx and increasing his mouth breathing. He had been using a great deal of unnecessary tension when reciting. This could be described as similar to someone grimacing as they tackle a task, or when exercising.

Shortening and tensing the neck increases tension in the whole organism and even affects concentration. Unfortunately we tend to tense up whenever we are faced with difficult situations, whether in our daily life or during sports and leisure activities.

Alexander found that he could release the tension in his neck but could not correct the laryngeal or respiratory problems. He surmised that the neck tension was causing the other problems, and suggested that the 'primary control' situated in the neck governed all the reflexes in the body. When this primary control is disturbed it can offset all the reflexes of the body and result in a lack of co-ordination and balance, leading to inefficiency in movement. This leads to a loss of form and can result in injury.

Alexander developed a system for releasing that tension, and taught others to do so. Now there are thousands of Alexander Technique teachers internationally.

Basic Alexander Technique

A fundamental principle of the Alexander Technique is that you do not 'do' the releasing and relaxation, but that you tell yourself what should be happening. In this way your head takes a position that is upward and forward, your neck relaxes and lengthens, your shoulders relax and widen and your back relaxes and lengthens. I repeat, do not 'do' all these, but repeat the following directions to yourself:

1) Head forward and upward.
2) Neck relax, neck lengthen.
3) Shoulders relax, shoulders lengthen.
4) Back relax, back lengthen.

Doing More

There are several excellent books on the Alexander Technique. Most of these will provide sufficient information for sports people to make use of the technique in their activities. If you feel that you would like to learn more about the technique, or if you have a serious back problem it is worthwhile consulting a qualified teacher.

I often recommend the Alexander Technique to back sufferers in my practice, usually with very encouraging results.

HYPNOTHERAPY

In recent years hypnotherapy has become a more popular form of complementary medicine and its full potential and benefits are still being explored. It is important to say that the use of hypnosis should only be carried out by competent and qualified therapists who are conscious of the psychological implications of the technique.

Hypnosis is a vehicle that allows the subconscious mind to be empowered by suggestion. It is certainly not a means by which one person 'controls' the mind of another, as is suggested by many stage hypnotists. Hypnotherapists suffer more than any of the complementary medicines from a distorted public image. They are serious and competent therapists who achieve wonderful results in appropriate conditions.

Enhancing Performance

For the purposes of this book, the potential for enhancing performance is the aspect of hypnotherapy which I wish to recommend. In modern terms, hypnotherapy can be used to develop 'focusing', 'centering' and a 'positive mental attitude' – the very qualities relevant to achieving enhanced sports performance.

Hypnotherapy can be used in three distinct areas: preparation, participation and follow-up.

Preparation is the most important of these, and takes the most time. It allows the sportsman to perform at the optimum level by eliminating all negative thoughts and replacing them with positive attitudes. The therapist may need to explore the athlete's life outside of sport to determine whether any problems in those areas might be affecting performance. It may be difficult to encourage a high level of skilled performance if the athlete's personal life is causing stressful reactions.

Preparation can be valuable for a sportsman to reach successive peaks during a long season or tournament. A golfer or snooker player, or participant in other sports needing a similar level of intense concentration, could use hypnotherapy to enable him to relax, focus and concentrate. A hypnotherapy treatment before the start of the season or tournament may be reinforced at appropriate times. The competitor can learn to recall embedded suggestions by using key words or actions as triggers.

Many performers learn to use visualisation and mental rehearsal techniques. A hypnotherapist can help the performer to create a set of pictures which he can use to rehearse and prepare for each match, and thus approach it in a positive way. Eliminating the negative constraints of the left hemisphere of the brain, for instance, often enables smoother intuitive right hemisphere performance.

The sportsman learns to refer to previous performances or patterns, to break them down into different sensory modes of sight, sound, smell, feelings, kinaesthetics and taste. When he has increased his awareness of these, the therapist helps him to build them into a total positive sensory experience which can be repeated many times and triggered at will.

During the participation phase the sportsman can trigger and access the stored resources in a positive way. Calm and relaxation can be induced during a waiting time so as to conserve energy and concentration, which can then be released as necessary.

Follow-up consists of re-running the event and continuing to build the positive visualisation. Healing and recreation can be enhanced by deep relaxation and suggestion, enabling the athlete to be ready for the next event in a refreshed and positive way.

Appendix I

Homoeopathic Suppliers and Organisations

Ainsworths Homoeopathic Pharmacy, 36 New Cavendish Street, London W1M 7LH, UK.

Biological Homeopathic Industries, 11600 Cochiti S.E., Albuquerque, NM 87123, USA.

Boericke and Tafel, 2381 Circadian Way, Santa Rosa, CA 95407, USA.

Boiron USA, 6 Campus Boulevard, Bldg A, Newtown Square, PA 19073, USA.

Brauer Biotherapies, P.O. Box 234, Tanunda 5352, Australia.

British Homoeopathic Association, 27A Devonshire Street, London W1N 1RJ, UK. (List of medical homoeopaths available on request.)

Dolisos USA, 3014 Rigel Avenue, Las Vegas, NV 89102, USA.

Faculty of Homoeopathy, 15 Clerkenwell Close, London EC1R 0AA, UK. (List of medical homoeopaths available on request.)

Faculty of Homoeopathy (Scotland), Glasgow Homoeopathic Hospital, 1053 Great Western Road, Glasgow G12 0XQ, UK.

Freeman's Homoeopathic Pharmacy, 20 Main Street, Busby, Glasgow G76 7DU, UK.

Helios Homoeopathic Pharmacy, 97 Camden Road, Tunbridge Wells TN1 2QR, UK.

Homoeopathic Educational Services, 2124 Kittredge Street, Berkeley, CA 94704, USA.

Homoeopathic Supply Co. (for dispensing containers, bottles etc.) Fairview, 4 Nelson Road, Sheringham, Norfolk NR26 8BU, UK.

Minimum Price Books, 250 H Street, P.O. Box 2187, Blaine, WA 98231, USA.

National Center for Homeopathy, 801 North Fairfax Street, Suite 306, Alexandria, VA 22314, USA.

Nelson's Homoeopathic Pharmacy, 15 Duke Street, Dublin 2, Ireland.

Nelson's Homoeopathic Pharmacy, 73 Duke Street, London W1M 6BY, UK.

Society of Homoeopaths, 2 Artizan Road, Northampton
NN1 4HU, UK. (List of professional homoeopaths available
on request.)

Standard Homeopathic Co., 210 West 131st Street, Los Angeles,
CA 90061, USA.

Thompsons Homeopathic Supplies, 844 Yonge Street, Toronto, Ont.
M4W 2H1, Canada.

Weleda (Ireland), Sroughan, Lacken, Blessington, Co. Wicklow,
Ireland.

Weleda (NZ), P.O. 8132, Te Mata Peak Road, Havelock North,
New Zealand.

Weleda (SA), P.O. 494, Bergvlei 2012, South Africa.

Weleda (UK), Heanor Road, Ilkeston, Derbyshire DE7 8DR, UK.

Weleda (USA), P.O. 249, Congers, NY 10920, USA.

Appendix II

Homoeopathic First Aid Kit

Unless otherwise stated all the remedies should be carried in tablet form. The 6c potency will usually be the most effective for first contact treatment.

Remedies

1) Antimonium Crudum
2) Arnica
3) Arsenicum Album
4) Belladonna
5) Bellis Perennis
6) Bryonia
7) Calendula (cream and lotion)
8) Calendula
9) Cantharis
10) Carbo Vegetabilis
11) Causticum
12) Cuprum
13) Glonoine
14) Hypericum
15) Kali Bichromicum
16) Ledum Palustre
17) Magnesium Phosphoricum
18) Natrum Sulphuricum
19) Rhus Toxicodendron
20) Ruta Graveolens
21) Urtica Urens (ointment)
22) Bach Rescue Remedy (liquid)

Appendix III

References and Further Reading

References

Barker H.B., Beynon B.D. & Renström A.F.H., 1997. *Sports Medicine* **23**, 2: 69–73

Bentley, J.D., 1996. *Sports Medicine* **22**, 3: 409–20

Brinson, P. & Dick, F., 1996. *Fit to Dance*, National Inquiry into Dancers' Health and Injury: 14, 47, 63, 106, 154

Cross, V. & Boivin, C. 1995. 'Bone density and injury in ballet dancers', *Dancing Times*: 1187–9

Davies, C.T.M. & Taylor, P., 1995. *Sports Medicine* **21**, 1: 1–6

Dreisinger, T. & Nelson, A.G., 1995. *Sports Medicine* **21**, 4: 313–20

Fowler, J.A., 1984. *Cash's Textbook of Orthopaedics and Rheumatology for Physiotherapists*: 512–52

Fredericson, J.A., 1996. *Sports Medicine* **21**, 1: 49–72

Galli, L., 1994. *Dance Magazine*: 68

Keay, N., 1995. 'Dancers, periods and osteoporosis', *Dancing Times*: 1189

Keene, J.S.,1990. *Orthopaedic and Sports Physiotherapy*

Jackson, D.W. et al., 1978. 'Injury prediction in the young athlete', *American Journal of Sports Medicine* **6**: 6–14

Lachman, S. & Jenner, J.R., 1992. *Soft Tissue Injuries in Sport*

O'Connor, P.J., Lewis, R.D. & Boyd, A., 1996. *Sports Medicine* **21**, 5: 321–5

Reider, B., 1996. *Sports Medicine* **21**, 2: 147–56

Sanderson, F.H., 1981. 'The psychology of the injury-prone athlete', *Sports Fitness and Sports Injuries*, Faber and Faber, London: 31–6

Shek, P.P. & Shepperd, R.J., 1994. *The Journal of Sports Medicine and Physical Fitness* **34**, 1: 11–19

Further Reading

The Alexander Technique, Richard Brennan. Element Books, ISBN 1–85230–217–8

Classical Homoeopathy, Margery Blackie. Beaconsfield Publishers, ISBN 0–906584–14–0

The Complete Homeopathy Handbook, Miranda Castro. Macmillan London, ISBN 0333–42888–9

Insights Into Homoeopathy, Frank Bodman. Beaconsfield Publishers, ISBN 0–906584–28–0

Fit to Dance? Peter Brinson & Fiona Dick. Calouste Gulbenkian Foundation (UK), ISBN 0–903319–70–5

The Lotus Materia Medica, Robin Murphy. Lotus Star Academy, ISBN 0–9635764–0–2

Phataks's Materia Medica of Homoeopathic Medicines, S. R. Phatak. Foxlee-Vaughan Publishers, ISBN 1–870292–01–4

Organon of the Medical Art, Samuel Hahnemann, Trans. Wenda Brewster O'Reilly. Birdcage Books, ISBN 1–889613–01–0

Portraits of Homeopathic Remedies, Catherine R. Coulter. North Atlantic Books, ISBN 1–55643–036–1

The Principles, Art and Practice of Homoeopathy, Trevor Smith. Insight Editions, ISBN 0–946670–07–2

Qi Gong for Health and Vitality, Michael Tse. Judy Piatkus (Publishers), ISBN 0–7499–1336–3

The Reflexology Handbook, Laura Norman with Thomas Cowan. Judy Piatkus (Publishers), ISBN 0–86188–912–6

The Science of Homeopathy, George Vithoulkas. Thorsons Publishing Group, ISBN 0–7225–1310–0

Soft Tissue Injuries in Sport, Sylvia Lachmann & John R. Jenner. Blackwell Scientific Publications, ISBN 0–632–03508–0

Sports and Exercise Injuries, Steven Subotnik. North Atlantic Books, ISBN 0–55643–114–7

Sports Injuries, Christopher M. Norris. Butterworth-Heinemann, ISBN 0–7506–0156–6

Sports Injuries, Vivian Grisogino. John Murray (Publishers), ISBN 0–7195–4111–5

Studies of Homoeopathic Remedies, Douglas M. Gibson. Beaconsfield Publishers, ISBN 0–906584–17–5

Synthesis: Repertorium Homeopathicum Syntheticum, Frederik Schroyens. Homeopathic Book Publishers & Archibel SA, ISBN 0–9522744–9–3

Tutorials on Homoeopathy, Donald Foubister. Beaconsfield Publishers, ISBN 0–906584–25–6

Remedy Index

General Index

abdomen, abdominal, 44, 63, 137,
   221, 222
  pain, 48, 49, 50, 133,
    in constipation, **187**, 188,
    with diarrhoea, **192**,
    extending from genitals, **137**
    from sacrum, **167**
  weakness in dancers, **163**
  wind, **204**
abduction,
  knee injury, from, **124**
  groin strain, in, **133**
  shoulder, **140**, 141, 142, 145, 229
abrasions, 47, **65**, 226
abscess, tooth, **209**, 246
absent-minded, 45, **278**, 279
accident, 24, 36, **65**, 158, 213, **216**,
   234, 241, 271
Achilles tendon, 90, **102**, 103, 224,
   228, 260, 261, 263, 264, 268
  crepitus, in, **103**
  rupture, **102**
  tendinitis, **103**
acromioclavicular sprain, **150**, 151,
   223, 229, 261
adductor, strain, **134**
adhesions, 98, **119**, 121, 257, 264
alcohol, **179**, 197, 200,
altitude, 5, **179**, 180, 193, 194, 231,
   286
  acclimatisation, to, **179**, 286
amenorrhoea, 74, **205**
  and periods, **205**
anger, 13, 26, 77, 204, 219, 223, 245,
   249, 266, 280
  injury, after, **277**, 279,
  nervous, **204**
ankle, 11, 12, 19, 25, 47, 52, 57, 81,
   94, 105, 114, 215, 217, 218,
   221, 223, 229, 242, 243, 244,
   257, 258, 260, 261, 264, 266,
   267

ankle (*continued*)
  fractures, 100
  injuries, **94**
  osteoarthritis, **104**
  sprains, **94**
  weak, **99**
ankylosing spondylitis, 40, 86
anticipation, 227, 232, 236, 283
  anxiety from, **288**
  diarrhoea, with, **202**
  nervous, 204, 237, 264,
  self-confidence, loss of, **186**
anus, 192, **206**, 248, 250, 251
  closed sensation, 188
  piles, **206**
anxiety, 2, 22, 71, **180**, 276, 279,
   280, 281, 283, 287, **288**, 289,
   301
  anticipation, **288**
  dancers, in, **2**, 22,
  fatigue, and, **71**
  stress, and, **287**
apathetic, **199**, 222, 230, 237, 251,
   279
  homesickness, in, **199**
  injury, after, **279**
apophysitis,
  calcaneal, 82, **89**
appetite, 232, 237
  heat stroke, with, 198
  loss at altitude, 179
  nausea, with, 202, 204, 205, 206
apprehension, 74, **270**
arthritis, 40, **104**, 223, 256, 257, 258
asthma, **180**, 190, 265
atrophy, 22, 59, **60**, 103, 216, 224

back pain, **162**, 164, 165, 170, 213,
   222, 247, 259, 261, 269
  as concomitant, 45
  extending from groin, 133
  lower, 162

NOTES

NOTES

NOTES

NOTES

Classical Homoeopathy, Dr Margery Blackie, 1986, reprinted 1990 with Repertory. The complete teaching legacy of one of the most important homoeopaths of our time.   0906584140

Comparative Materia Medica, Dr E. F. Candegabe, 1997. Detailed comparative study of thirty-seven remedies by one of the Argentinian masters.   0906584361

Everyday Homoeopathy (2nd Edition), Dr David Gemmell, 1997. A practical handbook for using homoeopathy in the context of one's own personal and family health care, using readily available remedies.

0906584442

Homoeopathic Prescribing, Dr Noel Pratt, revised 1985. A compact reference book covering 161 common complaints and disorders, with guidance on the choice of the appropriate remedy.   0906584035

Homoeopathic Treatment of Beef and Dairy Cattle, C. E. I. Day, MRCVS, 1995. Describes how homoeopathy may be used in the care of cattle, both as individuals and in a group.   090658437X

Homoeopathic Treatment of Eczema, Robin Logan, FSHom, 1998. A textbook on the homoeopathic treatment of this condition.

0906584477

Homoeopathy, Dr T. P. Paschero, (in production, 2000). Dr Paschero's major work on the subject.   0906584418

Homoeopathy as Art and Science, Dr Elizabeth Wright Hubbard, 1990. The selected writings of one of the foremost modern homoeopaths.   0906584264

Homoeopathy in Practice, Dr Douglas Borland, 1982, reprinted 1988 with Symptom Index. Detailed guidance on the observation of symptoms and the choice of remedies.   090658406X

Homoeopathy for Sports, Exercise and Dance, Emlyn Thomas, DPhysEd, RSHom, 1999. A practical handbook for sports medicine practitioners, coaches, teachers, players and dancers.   0906584485

In Search of the Later Hahnemann, Rima Handley, DPhil, FSHom, 1997. A study of Hahnemann's practice in Paris, with material from his casebooks of that period.   0906584353

Insights into Homoeopathy, Dr Frank Bodman, 1990. Homoeopathic approaches to common problems in general medicine and psychiatry.

0906584280

(*continued overleaf*)

(*continued from previous page*)

Introduction to Homoeopathic Medicine (2nd Edition), Dr Hamish Boyd, 1989. A formal introductory text, written in categories familiar to the medical practitioner.   0906584213

Materia Medica of New Homoeopathic Remedies, Dr O. A. Julian, paperback edition 1984. Full clinical coverage of 106 new homoeopathic remedies, for use in conjunction with the classical materia medicas.   0906584116

Mental Symptoms in Homoeopathy, Dr Luis Detinis, 1994. A comparative study of the Mind rubrics in Kent's *Repertory*.   0906584345

Studies of Homoeopathic Remedies, Dr Douglas Gibson, 1987. Detailed clinical studies of 100 major remedies. Well-known for the uniquely wide range of insights brought to bear on each remedy.
                                                        0906584175

Tutorials on Homoeopathy, Dr Donald Foubister, 1989. Detailed studies on a wide range of conditions and remedies.   0906584256

Typology in Homoeopathy, Dr Léon Vannier, 1992. A study of human types, based on the gods of Antiquity and the remedies which are relevant to them.   0906584302